Research Progress in Alzheimer's Disease and Dementia

Dementia, Diabetes, and Hypertension

Is There a Unified Theory through a Dysregulation of the Ca^{2+} Homeostasis?

RESEARCH PROGRESS IN ALZHEIMER'S DISEASE AND DEMENTIA

Additional books and e-books in this series can be found on Nova's website under the Series tab.

RESEARCH PROGRESS IN ALZHEIMER'S DISEASE AND DEMENTIA

DEMENTIA, DIABETES, AND HYPERTENSION

IS THERE A UNIFIED THEORY THROUGH A DYSREGULATION OF THE CA^{2+} HOMEOSTASIS?

LEANDRO BUENO BERGANTIN

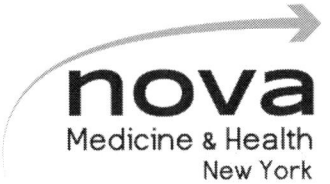

Copyright © 2021 by Nova Science Publishers, Inc.

All rights reserved. No part of this book may be reproduced, stored in a retrieval system or transmitted in any form or by any means: electronic, electrostatic, magnetic, tape, mechanical photocopying, recording or otherwise without the written permission of the Publisher.

We have partnered with Copyright Clearance Center to make it easy for you to obtain permissions to reuse content from this publication. Simply navigate to this publication's page on Nova's website and locate the "Get Permission" button below the title description. This button is linked directly to the title's permission page on copyright.com. Alternatively, you can visit copyright.com and search by title, ISBN, or ISSN.

For further questions about using the service on copyright.com, please contact:
Copyright Clearance Center
Phone: +1-(978) 750-8400   Fax: +1-(978) 750-4470   E-mail: info@copyright.com.

NOTICE TO THE READER

The Publisher has taken reasonable care in the preparation of this book, but makes no expressed or implied warranty of any kind and assumes no responsibility for any errors or omissions. No liability is assumed for incidental or consequential damages in connection with or arising out of information contained in this book. The Publisher shall not be liable for any special, consequential, or exemplary damages resulting, in whole or in part, from the readers' use of, or reliance upon, this material. Any parts of this book based on government reports are so indicated and copyright is claimed for those parts to the extent applicable to compilations of such works.

Independent verification should be sought for any data, advice or recommendations contained in this book. In addition, no responsibility is assumed by the publisher for any injury and/or damage to persons or property arising from any methods, products, instructions, ideas or otherwise contained in this publication.

This publication is designed to provide accurate and authoritative information with regard to the subject matter covered herein. It is sold with the clear understanding that the Publisher is not engaged in rendering legal or any other professional services. If legal or any other expert assistance is required, the services of a competent person should be sought. FROM A DECLARATION OF PARTICIPANTS JOINTLY ADOPTED BY A COMMITTEE OF THE AMERICAN BAR ASSOCIATION AND A COMMITTEE OF PUBLISHERS.

Additional color graphics may be available in the e-book version of this book.

Library of Congress Cataloging-in-Publication Data

ISBN: 978-1-53619-227-8

Published by Nova Science Publishers, Inc. † New York

*I dedicate this book to my parents Maria Lúcia
and Armando Magno (in memoriam).
I also dedicate this book to my aunt Maria de Fátima,
to my grandparents Maria Emília and José Bueno (in memoriam),
and to my brother Lucas.*

Contents

Preface		xi
Acknowledgments		xiii
Abbreviations		xv
Chapter 1	Introduction	1
Chapter 2	Importance of the Exocytosis Study for the Neurotransmitters and Hormones Release: Fundamental Findings for Understanding Neurological and Psychiatric Diseases	15
Chapter 3	Ca^{2+} Signalling Involved in the Exocytosis of Neuroendocrine Cells: Basic Concepts for Understanding Neurological and Psychiatric Diseases	19
Chapter 4	Role of cAMP in the Exocytosis of the Neuroendocrine Cells: Fundamental Concepts for Studying Neurological and Psychiatric Diseases	31
Chapter 5	Novel Concepts from the Ca^{2+}/cAMP Interaction: Impact in Neurological and Psychiatric Diseases	39

Chapter 6	The Pharmacological Modulation of the Ca^{2+}/cAMP Signalling Interaction as a Therapeutic Strategy for Neurological and Psychiatric Diseases: A Theory and Supporting Data	65
Chapter 7	Paradoxical Effects of the CCB and Their Pleiotropic Effects	73
Chapter 8	Additional Interesting Findings, and Concepts, for the Ca^{2+}/cAMP Signalling Pathways and Neurological/Psychiatric Disorders Field	77
Chapter 9	Hypertension and Higher Risk for the Decline of Cognition	93
Chapter 10	Hypertension and Higher Risk for Diabetes	97
Chapter 11	A Link between Diabetes and Dementia	101
Chapter 12	Synopsis	105
Chapter 13	Future Directions	107
Chapter 14	Conclusion	111
Bibliography		115
About the Author		151
Index		153

"In that rainy afternoon, the young researcher and his supervisor were preparing their daily experiment. On its course, there was a remaining solution containing Verapamil, a classical L-type CCB. In a relapse, the young researcher decided to add this solution (containing CCB) in an isolated smooth muscle. There was no apparent reason for it! The smooth muscle was prior relaxed with a drug (rolipram) that increased the cAMP cytosolic concentration. Putatively, addition of verapamil in the isolated smooth muscle should enhance (much more) the relaxation of the muscle contractions sympathetically mediated! To his surprise, it was like that: the young researcher witnessed a drastic contraction of the smooth muscle! Puzzled with what he had observed, the young researcher and his supervisor did not know the impact and the magnitude of their discovery until that time"

PREFACE

Dementia, diabetes, and hypertension are considered huge medical problems around the world, costing many millions of dollars to the medical health systems. Curiously, hypertension has been clinically linked with a higher risk for decline of cognition, as shown in dementia patients. In addition, there is a clear clinical association between hypertension and diabetes, reflecting substantial similarities in their etiology. In fact, consistent data support that patients diagnosed with diabetes have shown an increased risk of presenting cognitive dysfunctions, clinical signs of dementia. Considering the cumulative knowledge from the scientific literature, we can now link Ca^{2+} signals dysregulations as an upstream issue for hypertension, diabetes and other inflammatory processes, and dementia. Regarding therapeutics, hypertensive patients have been classically treated with Ca^{2+} channel blockers (CCBs), medicines whose mechanism of action consists in reducing the influx of Ca^{2+} into the cells. Intriguingly, many clinical reports have been demonstrating off-label effects for CCBs. In hypertensive patients treated with CCBs, it can be observed a lower incidence of dementia such as Alzheimer's disease. The possible mechanism of action could be attributed to a restoration of the Ca^{2+} homeostasis. In addition, in hypertensive patients treated with CCBs, it can be also observed an improvement of diabetes status such as glycemic control. A possible mechanism of action could be due to a restoration of insulin secretion, then achieving glycemic control, and a reduction of the pancreatic β-cell apoptosis. Thus, this book puts together fundamental concepts, and current therapies to treat dementia, hypertension, and diabetes, including novel therapeutics coming from the pharmacological manipulation of Ca^{2+}/cAMP signalling. Finally, this book compiles more than 300 references from the scientific literature, including data of high evidence such as meta-analysis and systematic reviews, and discusses pharmaceuticals already approved and clinically safe, e.g., CCBs, then allowing sustained increments in the life quality of age-related patients.

ACKNOWLEDGMENTS

Thanks to Nova Science Publishers for releasing this book.

ABBREVIATIONS

AC	adenylyl cyclases
ACh	acetylcholine
AD	Alzheimer's disease
ALS	Amyotrophic Lateral Sclerosis
BAY	K 8644 Ca^{2+} channels activator
BP	blood pressure
Ca^{2+}	calcium ion
CCB/CCBs	Ca^{2+} channel blockers
CICR	Ca^{2+}-induced Ca^{2+}-release
ER	endoplasmic reticulum
HD	Huntington´s disease
IBMX	3-isobutyl-1-methylxanthine
IP_3R	inositol trisphosphate receptor
IRBIT	IP_3R binding protein released with IP3
LDCV	large dense-core vesicle
MIT	mitochondria
NA	noradrenaline
NCX	Na^+/Ca^{2+} exchanger
PD	Parkinson's disease
PDE	phosphodiesterases
PKA	protein kinase cAMP-dependent

PKC	protein kinase Ca^{2+}-dependent
RRP	ready-release-vesicle-pool
RyR	ryanodine receptors
SERCA	sarcoendoplasmic Ca^{2+}-ATPase
SHR	spontaneously hypertensive rats
SMA	Spinal muscular atrophy
SQ 22536	adenylyl cyclase inhibitor
SV	synaptic vesicles
T2DM	type 2 diabetes mellitus
VACC/VACCs	voltage activated Ca^{2+} channels
VD	vascular dementia

Chapter 1

INTRODUCTION

Analyzing Medline database from 1975 to 1996, Grossman and Messerli [1] found 63 clinical studies, involving 1,252 hypertensive patients, reporting alterations of the sympathetic activity produced by an acute and chronic administration of the L-type calcium [Ca^{2+}] channel blockers (CCB or pharmacologically known as voltage-activated Ca^{2+} channels (VACC) blockers such as verapamil, diltiazem and nifedipine: important class of drugs largely used for the antihypertensive therapy by decreasing the arterial pressure due to the reduction of Ca^{2+} entry both into the cardiac and smooth muscle cells, and into the sympathetic neurons). Grossman and Messerli's study [1] showed that the acute administration of the CCB positively produced a significant reduction of the mean arterial pressure, but negatively produced a significant increment of plasma noradrenaline (NA) levels [sympathetic hyperactivity], and an increase of heart rate. This study showed that these adverse effects of the CCB (sympathetic hyperactivity) could be directly involved in the increase into morbidity, and mortality, associated to the chronic use of these drugs. However, the cellular and molecular mechanisms involved in this CCB-induced sympathetic hyperactivity remained unclear for several decades, or even more!

Using tissues richly innervated by sympathetic nerves as an *ex vivo* study model of the sympathetic neurotransmission, such as rodent vas deferens [2-7], several studies showed that verapamil produced paradoxical effects on the electrically-evoked neurogenic contractions mediated by the sympathetic nerves [8, 9]. These studies showed that in concentrations above 1 µM, verapamil inhibited these neurogenic contractions, but paradoxically potentiated these contractions in concentrations below 1 µM [10-13].

In fact, since 1975 it was reported that, despite the well-known effect of verapamil to block the sympathetically mediated contractions of the smooth muscles (vas deferens), lower concentrations of verapamil caused a surprising augmentation of those contractions [10]. In agreement with this, French & Scott (1981) [11] observed that verapamil unexpectedly potentiated the neurogenic contractions in the prostatic portion of vas deferens, but antagonized those of the epididymal portion. These authors provided no reasonable explanation for this paradoxical finding. Furthermore, six years later [12], another study reported that verapamil and diltiazem enhanced the purinergic-mediated neurogenic twitch responses of the electrically-stimulated rat vas deferens; the authors attributed this effect to an unrealistic agonist effect of verapamil on the presynaptic L-type VACC, thus enhancing the Ca^{2+} entry and the ATP release [12]. From these reports, we may already suggest that this paradoxical effect relies on increases in the secretory activity (response) of the sympathetic nerves. Two years later (1989), a fourth study appeared showing that both, L-type VACC blockers and activator BAY K 8644, elicited similar augmentations of the sympathetic contractions of the entire electrically-stimulated mouse vas deferens [13]. Most interesting, these authors observed that verapamil (30 µM) markedly enhanced the potentiation caused by Bay K 8644 in a supra-additive fashion, suggesting that verapamil and Bay K 8644 can enhance the neurogenic contractions by different mechanisms, discrediting the hypothesis of an agonist effect of verapamil on the presynaptic L-type VACC.

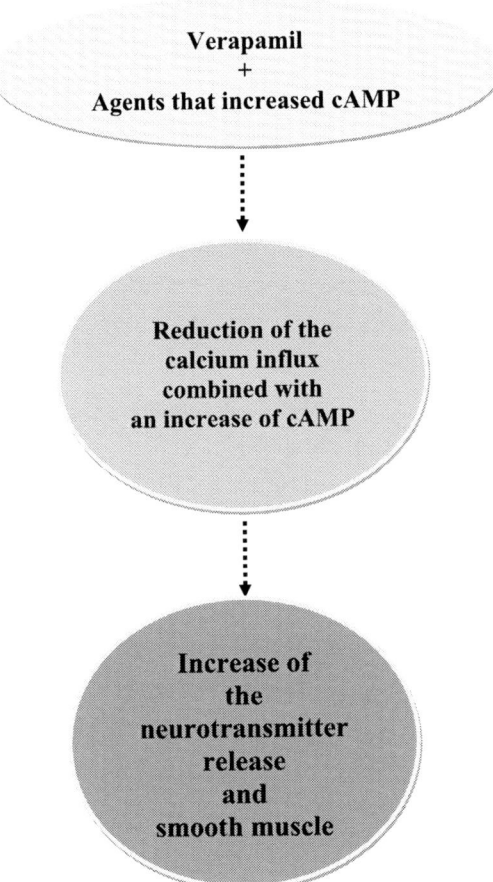

Figure 1.1. Effect of verapamil and agents that increased (cAMP)c (rolipram, IBMX and forskolin) on the neurogenic contractions mediated by the sympathetic nerves in rat vas deferens. Verapamil, in high concentrations (>10-6 M), inhibited neurogenic contractions due to the reduction of neurotransmitter release, but discreetly potentiated these contractions in low concentrations (<10-6 M). Pre-incubation of tissue (15 min) with agents that increased (cAMP) reversed verapamil inhibitory effect, resulting into potentiating neurogenic contractions. According to theoretical model proposed by Bergantin, the reduction of the calcium influx due to the L-type VACC blocker (verapamil), combined with an increase of cAMP, resulted in an increase of the neurotransmitter release from the sympathetic nerves of vas deferens.

In a recent study from our laboratory (see Figure 1.1), we could reproduce those earlier observations in the neurogenically-induced contractions of the rat vas deferens: at lower concentrations, verapamil elicited a tiny augmentation, while at higher concentrations the VACC blocker caused a full inhibition of the contractions [6, 14, 15]. The interesting finding was that, as the high verapamil concentrations, various cAMP enhancers such as phosphodiesterase (PDE) inhibitors, rolipram and IBMX (isobutyl methyl xanthine), and adenylyl cyclase (AC) activator forskolin, depressed the neurogenic vas deferens contractions; however, in the presence of cAMP enhancers, the lower concentrations of verapamil caused a drastic augmentation of the neurogenic contractions mediated by the endogenously released ATP. The inhibition of AC by SQ 22536 attenuated the enhanced contractions, suggesting that an interaction of the Ca^{2+}/cAMP intracellular signalling pathways (Ca^{2+}/cAMP interaction) could, perhaps, explain the paradoxical effects of the combined drugs, verapamil and cAMP enhancers [6].

On the basis of the classical receptor theory, the combination of two drugs with an inhibitory action produces inhibitory effects [16]. Thus, the potentiation of the neurogenic contractions of the rat vas deferens by a simultaneous administration of verapamil and (cAMP)c enhancers is an experimental finding unexpected in accordance with the receptor theory. The interaction between the intracellular signalling pathways mediated by cAMP and Ca^{2+} could explain in a more consistent way this pharmacological phenomenon. The idea of this interaction was supported by various experimental protocols.

Bergantin et al. [6] showed that the potentiation of the smooth muscles neurogenic contractions produced by the combination of verapamil, and enhancers of cAMP cytosolic concentration ((cAMP)c), was prevented by a reduction of (cAMP)c caused by the AC inhibitor SQ 22536, or by depletion of the Ca^{2+} storages from the endoplasmic reticulum (ER) by the sarcoplasmic ER Ca^{2+} reuptake blocker thapsigargin [6]. These findings suggest that a blockade of the Ca^{2+} influx through the L-type CCB, by verapamil, produces a reduction of $(Ca^{2+})c$, leading into the increase of AC activity, that in turn results in an increase of (cAMP)c. The increase of (cAMP)c stimulates the Ca^{2+} release from the ER, and consequently increments cellular responses, as shown in Figure 1.2.

secretion [22] could also be explained in the context of the "calcium paradox." At higher concentrations, the intensive Ca^{2+} influx promoted by BAY K 8644 may inhibit the constitutive activity of the Ca^{2+} and cAMP signalling pathways associated to the L-type VACC, thus reducing the secretory response mediated by a Ca^{2+} release from the ER (Figure 1.2).

The concept of the complex cAMP-IP_3R interaction as a "third messenger," which may mediate the synergistic action of the Ca^{2+} and cAMP signalling, is now emerging [23]. Recent data suggest that IRBIT (Inositol-trisphosphate (IP_3) receptors binding protein released with IP3) may become a central-stage in the mechanism mediating the synergism between cAMP and Ca^{2+} signalling pathways, by functioning as a "third messenger," which favors the crosstalk between IP_3R and other proteins. Another central component is the classical phosphorylation by the protein kinase cAMP-dependent (PKA) of IP_3R. Thus, IP_3Rs, IRBIT, PKA and the effector proteins have to be assembled into microdomains to allow the efficiency of IRBIT. In resting cells, when cellular IP_3 levels are low, IRBIT is bound to the IP_3R; thus IP_3R functions to buffer the availability of free IRBIT [23]. Increases in cAMP levels may lead into the dissociation of IRBIT from IP_3 receptors, and its translocation into effector proteins located either at intracellular organelles and/or the plasma membrane; in this manner, IRBIT functions as a "third messenger" that transmits the information carried out by the second messengers cAMP and IP_3. At the same time, IRBIT integrates and synergizes the activity of the cAMP and Ca^{2+} signalling systems, providing a molecular mechanism for the synergistic action between them. We think this "idea" fits into the "calcium paradox" hypothesis; in fact, Ca^{2+} release from the ER into the cytosol, triggered by verapamil plus rolipram in rat chromaffin cell slices, was blocked upon an ER Ca^{2+} depletion with thapsigargin [6]. Furthermore, considering that this "calcium paradox" could also explain data from different biological systems [24, 25], it is becoming apparent that the enigma of the "calcium paradox" in the context of neurotransmission, and neurosecretion, may be resolved through the Ca^{2+}/cAMP interaction. However, further work is needed to clarify this challenging hypothesis.

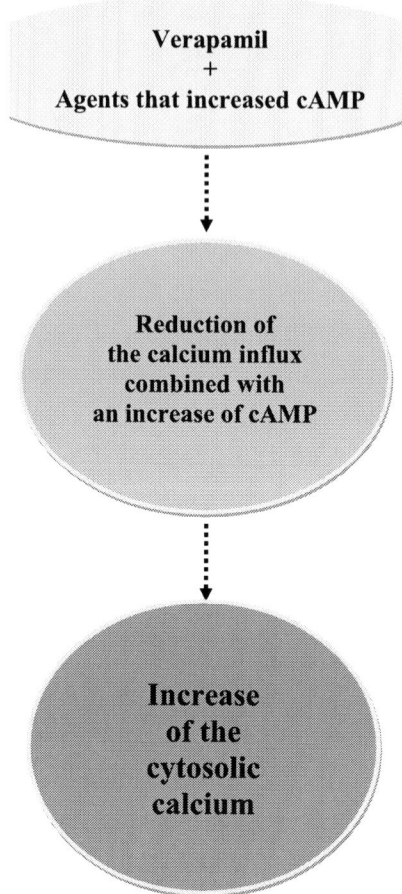

Figure 1.3 Effect of verapamil and rolipram on fluorescence associated to Ca^{2+} indicator (fura-2) in adrenal medullar slices. Verapamil reduced fluorescence unit by a reduction of Ca^{2+} influx due to the L-type VACC blocker. However, the pre-incubation of slices with rolipram produced a reversed effect of the verapamil effect, resulting into an increase of fura-2 fluorescence. Thapsigargin abolished this effect, indicating that the endoplasmic reticulum participates in this mechanism. According to the theoretical model proposed by Bergantin, the reduction of calcium influx due to the L-type VACC blocker (verapamil) combined with an increase of cAMP, due to a PDE inhibition (rolipram), resulted in an increase of catecholamine release from adrenal chromaffin cells due to an increase of Ca^{2+} cytosolic transients.

As in vas deferens, some paradoxical effects have also been recently reported to occur in adrenal chromaffin cells, another interesting model of neuroendocrine cell. For instance, in a study performed in voltage-clamped bovine chromaffin cells, the blockade of the L-type VACC with nifedipine transformed the exocytotic responses, elicited by a double-pulse protocol, from a depression into a facilitation [20]. In an earlier study, it was shown that nifedipine suppressed the endocytotic response triggered by a long depolarizing stimulus [26]. The explanation for the paradoxical effect of nifedipine could rest in the fact that the inhibition of a rapid endocytosis triggered by Ca^{2+} entry, through the L-type VACC of bovine chromaffin cells (α_{1D}, Cav 1.3), could unmask a full exocytotic response. A second explanation may lay in the observation that a Ca^{2+} entry through L-type VACC causes the inhibition of P/Q type VACC (α_{1A}, Cav 2.1) [27], that in chromaffin cells greatly contribute to the control of the secretory response [28]. By blocking the L-type VACC, nifedipine could remove the Ca^{2+} dependent inactivation of P/Q-type VACC to enhance a Ca^{2+} entry through them, and thereby augmenting the secretory response.

An additional explanation for the nifedipine paradoxical effect in chromaffin cells [20] could be found in the context of the "calcium paradox" described in the vas deferens, and in the Ca^{2+}/cAMP interaction [6]. In agreement with these observations, recent reports [29, 30] have observed an inhibitory effect of an extracellular Ca^{2+} on Ca^{2+} - dependent exocytosis. These apparent paradoxical findings may be explained in the context of the "calcium paradox" described in the vas deferens, and in the Ca^{2+}/cAMP interaction [6] (see Figure 1.3).

Thus, in the light of the paradoxical effects of the combined drugs, verapamil plus rolipram in the vas deferens, it could be possible to implicate cAMP also in the paradoxical effects of nifedipine in the secretory response of chromaffin cells. In fact, several reports have been published on the role of cAMP in the regulation of neurotransmitter release, as well as in the postsynaptic actions of different neurotransmitters [7]. Additionally, the release of sympathetic transmitters is regulated both by Ca^{2+} and cAMP [31-35]. For example, in 1987 Morita and colleagues [36] observed that forskolin enhanced both norepinephrine and endogenous catecholamine release evoked by 30 mM K^+ from chromaffin cells. The effects of forskolin were substantial when catecholamine release was evoked with low concentrations of acetylcholine (Ach), or excess of K^+. Forskolin also enhanced the catecholamine release induced by ionomycin and veratrine, or by caffeine in Ca^{2+}-free medium. The potentiation by forskolin of the ACh-evoked catecholamine release was manifested in low Ca^{2+} concentrations in the medium but decreased when Ca^{2+} concentration was increased. These results clearly do not respect the concept that the mitigation of a Ca^{2+} entry produced by CCB and/or decreased of Ca^{2+} medium concentration causes a diminution of cellular responses [37, 38]. Finally, these authors [39] suggested that cAMP could increase the stimulation-induced catecholamine release by enhancing the Ca^{2+} uptake across the plasma membrane and/or altering the Ca^{2+} flux in an intracellular Ca^{2+} store.

In this point of view, some studies have also shown a positive correlation between an elevation of $(cAMP)_c$ and the catecholamine release in bovine chromaffin cells, stimulated with nicotine [40], PACAP [41], histamine [42] or VIP [43]; this is also true for the PDE inhibitors rolipram or IBMX [44-46].

To enhance the secretion, cAMP may act at several targets, including the VACC of chromaffin cells, the regulation of the size of subplasmalemmal vesicle pools and/or the kinetics of the fusion pore during the last steps of exocytosis [44]. It is well established that the L-type VACC is the most sensitive to cAMP and PKA [47-49]. For example, in mouse chromaffin cells, rolipram augments both $(cAMP)_c$, L-currents and the secretion [18]. Also, rolipram increased the size of the ready-release-vesicle-pool (RRP) [50] by 75%, nearly doubled the membrane area of single vesicles in rat chromaffin cells [48], and augmented the quantal size by 38% also in rat chromaffin cells [51]. Furthermore, the AC activator forskolin enhanced by 50%, and rolipram by 25% the quantal size of single vesicles in bovine chromaffin cells [44]. On the other hand, in mouse chromaffin cells, rolipram increased more the size of the RRP [47%] than the quantity of Ca^{2+} penetrating into the cell [16%]; this suggests that about 30% of the increased secretion is Ca^{2+}-independent and occurs down-stream of a $(Ca2+)c$ elevation through the L-type VACC, most likely by affecting directly the secretory apparatus [18]. However, as in the vas deferens, Ca^{2+}/cAMP interaction may also occur in chromaffin cells; an evidence for such interaction is still actually lacking. Whether the paradoxical effects of nifedipine could be explained in the context of the "calcium paradox," emanated from the vas deferens, deserves more experimental attention. Dysregulation of this Ca^{2+}/cAMP interaction could lead into serious pathological consequences, such as cardiovascular dysfunctions.

Stressful situations like fear, cold, severe hypoglycemia, hemorrhage, and acute myocardial infarction trigger the release of neurotransmitters from postganglionic sympathetic neurons (ATP and noradrenaline) and hormones from chromaffin cells of adrenal medulla (ATP and adrenaline), which activate specific receptors located on the surface of effectors cells (smooth and cardiac muscles, and exocrine cells), stimulating the coordinated physiological response that prepares mammals' body to survive by combating an enemy, or to flee from danger. Firstly described as *"fight or flight"* responses by American physiologist Walter Bradford Cannon at the beginning of the twentieth century [52], these physiological reactions to stress mediated by the sympathetic nervous system, and controlled by the central nervous system nuclei at the cortex, hypothalamus and spinal cord are vital to the survival of mammals, including humans. Thus, the heart rate, the strength of myocardial contraction and blood pressure increase; the blood flow switches into the skeletal muscle; glucose is mobilized from the liver and rises into the circulation; and the pupils and bronchioles dilate [52].

Several experimental and clinical studies, performed since 1950 decade, have shown that alterations in the activity of sympathoadrenal axis, and the subsequent rate of catecholamine release, are involved in the pathogenesis of the cardiovascular diseases, including systemic arterial hypertension in humans and in animal models, such as *Spontaneously Hypertensive Rats* (SHR) [53-57]. For example, a sympathetic hyperactivity characterized by a significant elevation of circulating levels of noradrenaline, and adrenaline, due to catecholamines hypersecretion by medullary adrenal tumor is involved in the severe hypertensive crisis in humans with pheochromocytoma (malign tumor of adrenal medulla) [57]. A similar sympathetic hyperactivity due to catecholamines hypersecretion by sympathetic neurons, and adrenal chromaffin cells, is involved in the pathogenesis of primary hypertension in humans and SHR [54-56]. Although a catecholamine hypersecretion from sympathetic neurons, and adrenal chromaffin cells, constitutes a primary dysfunction responsible by arterial hypertension; and that the use of drugs that interfere with sympathoadrenal axis, such as blockers of α- and β-adrenoceptors, constitutes a classical strategy to treat human hypertension; the cellular and molecular mechanisms involved in this sympathetic dysfunction are yet unclear.

Due to the common embryologic origin with postganglionic sympathetic neurons in the neural crest [58], the adrenal chromaffin cells are of interest not only as the basis of the *"fight or flight"* response and sympathetic dysfunctions, but also because they have been excellent models to study the working of other secretory cells. Because of their unlimited availability, particularly from bovine species, and their ease of isolation and preparation in primary cultures [59], chromaffin cells have been widely used in biochemical, electrophysiological, and neuropharmacological studies. Their usefulness has been further enhanced by the development of techniques to separate noradrenaline- from adrenaline-containing vesicles [60, 61]. Thus, fundamental findings on the catecholamine synthesis, storage, and release were extrapolated, with success, from these cells into basic neurotransmission mechanisms in the central and peripheral nervous systems.

Although the *"fight or flight"* response is complex, this response basically depends on a release of neurotransmitters, and hormones, synthesized and stored by postganglionic sympathetic neurons and adrenal chromaffin cells [52]. The physiological function of the chromaffin cells consists in the exocytotic release of the catecholamines (noradrenaline and adrenaline) into the circulation in response to stressor stimuli [62]. But, the demonstration that this secretory response was suppressed in the absence of extracellular Ca^{2+} became a clear notion that the release of hormone from neuroendocrine cells, and neurotransmitter from neurons, is tightly regulated with exocytotic fusion of secretory vesicles being triggered by a rise in $(Ca^{2+})_c$ [50, 63].

Because the exocytosis is a Ca^{2+}-dependent process [63], it is not surprising that chromaffin cells have been widely used as models to study the correlation between Ca^{2+} and exocytosis [50]. They contain all the elements required for a strict control, both spatial and kinetic, of the Ca^{2+} transients required during the various steps of exocytosis in neuronal and endocrine cells [64]. Adrenal chromaffin cells and postganglionic sympathetic neurons are excitable cells, which fire action potentials, opening plasmalemmal VACC, producing a Ca^{2+} entry into the cytosol, an increase of both $(Ca^{2+})_c$ and the exocytosis [65-68]. Because cytoplasmic organelles can take up and release Ca^{2+} into the cytosol, understanding the cytosolic Ca^{2+} signal requires the understanding of the Ca^{2+} redistribution between the cytosol and the different organelles [14, 69-71].

The development of high resolution methodologies for the study of Ca^{2+} signals in the live cells has produced important advances in the understanding of Ca^{2+} redistribution between the cytosol, and in the different organelles in neurons and neuroendocrine cells. For example, the manipulation of photoprotein aequorin genes [72, 73] has made it possible to introduce targeting sequences and to measure selective $(Ca^{2+})_c$ changes in different cytoplasmic organelles, allowing to study the precise role of these organelles in shaping Ca^{2+} signalling and in the exocytosis [71-79].

Some studies suggest that various intracellular messengers can participate in shaping Ca^{2+} signalling and exocytosis in neurons and neuroendocrine cells, including inositol triphosphate (IP_3) and protein kinase C (PKC) [80-84]. It was shown that cAMP can increase the transmitter release at many synapses in the autonomic nervous system of vertebrates, including sympathetic [80, 81] and parasympathetic ganglion neurons [82], and yet increases the catecholamines secretion from adrenal chromaffin cells [41, 43, 83, 84]. Although the cellular and molecular mechanisms involved in these facilitatory actions of cAMP on the exocytosis of neurotransmitter and hormones are unclear, the evidences suggest that this intracellular messenger can thus participate in the fine regulation of the exocytosis due to its modulatory action on the intracellular Ca^{2+} signals.

Based on the discovery of the involvement of the "*calcium paradox*" in the regulation of sympathetic neurotransmission by Bergantin and collaborators in 2013 [6], in which the interaction between Ca^{2+} and cAMP intracellular signalling pathways can finely modulate the neurotransmitter release from sympathetic neurons, and hormone secretion from adrenal chromaffin cells, we discussed in this book the role of this interaction in the physiological regulation of sympathetic activity, and its possible implications in the sympathetic dysfunctions related to the cardiovascular and other diseases, and yet benefits and risks of its pharmacological manipulation.

Chapter 2

IMPORTANCE OF THE EXOCYTOSIS STUDY FOR THE NEUROTRANSMITTERS AND HORMONES RELEASE: FUNDAMENTAL FINDINGS FOR UNDERSTANDING NEUROLOGICAL AND PSYCHIATRIC DISEASES

In general, the cellular communication involves a series of codes that combine electrical (action potentials) and chemical (neurotransmitters and neuromodulators) signals. The chemical signals depend of biosynthesis, storage, secretion, action in receptors and enzymatic degradation of neurotransmitters and hormones. Exocytosis constitutes the main cellular mechanism for secreting the neurotransmitters and hormones stored in secretory vesicles, or granules. It entails the fusion of secretory vesicle with the plasmalemma, thus promoting the release of its soluble content into the extracellular space. Exocytosis gave support to the classical quantal theory, which reinforces that neurotransmitters are released as discrete packages from the nerve terminals towards the postsynaptic cell.

A great part of the molecular structure of the secretory machine is known to be responsible for a fast neurotransmitter release at the synapse, in response to the action potentials. Among the cell models that have provided insight into the molecular machine underlying the successive steps of exocytosis, chromaffin cells from the adrenal medulla have taken a prominent place. These neuroendocrine cells are ideally suited to distinguish and quantify the diverse pools of vesicles [85, 86]. These cells, like postganglionic sympathetic neurons, are derived from the neural crest and receive cholinergic input from the preganglionic neurons of the splanchnic nerve. Since they also are excitable cells that generate action potentials, chromaffin cells are viewed as the endocrine counterparts of postganglionic sympathetic neurons, and are often termed adrenal paraneurons [87, 88].

It has been known that the sympathetic activation of chromaffin cells releases their hormones into the bloodstream in a Ca^{2+}-dependent manner. In addition, large dense-core vesicle (LDCV) exocytosis from adrenal chromaffin cells shares many important features with the neurotransmitter release from the synaptic vesicles (SV) in classical central nervous system synapses. Both are Ca^{2+}-dependent processes and are blocked by the action of neurotoxins, including tetanus and botulinum toxins. The phenomena of the two maturation steps preceding fusion, docking, and priming, are readily demonstrated in both neurons and chromaffin cells, and the release occurs from RRP. This release is carried out for the most part by proteins identical or very similar to those functioning at the synapses [89]. A series of proteins that act as part of a conserved core machinery for the vesicle docking and fusion throughout the cell have been identified. In regulated exocytosis, this core machinery must be controlled by Ca^{2+}-sensor proteins that allow a rapid activation of the fusion process following an elevation of $(Ca^{2+})c$.

The pioneering work of Katz and collaborators in the early 1950s has demonstrated that an increase in $(Ca^{2+})c$ is the immediate trigger for neurotransmitters/hormones release from neurons, and neuroendocrine cells. Physiologically, this increase of $(Ca^{2+})c$ is primarily started by an activation of nicotinic cholinergic receptors on the surface of the neuronal body of postganglionic sympathetic neurons, and adrenal chromaffin cells by ACh from ending nerves of preganglionic neurons, derived from the thoracolumbar portion of medulla [90, 91]. In the adrenal chromaffin cells, this event triggers the release of adrenaline and noradrenaline from adrenal chromaffin cells into the bloodstream [89-93]. In the postganglionic sympathetic neurons, this event triggers the release of noradrenaline into the sympathetic neuro-effector synapses [89-93]. In these synapses, the adrenaline and noradrenaline interact with adrenoceptors on the surface of effector cells (smooth and cardiac muscle cells, and exocrine cells) producing a series of physiological reactions characterized as "*fight or flight*" responses, such as an elevation of blood pressure, acceleration of heart rate and hyperglycemia [52].

In mammals, the catecholamines synthesized by the adrenal chromaffin cells (adrenaline and noradrenaline) are storage in LDCV with a diameter of about 120 nm [94-96]. In LDCV and SV of sympathetic neurons, the catecholamines are stored and released by exocytosis together with several substances, including ATP, neuropeptide Y, enkephalins, chromogranins and others [87, 88]. There are two major types of regulated exocytosis: LDCV exocytosis (neuroendocrine, endocrine and exocrine cells) and SV exocytosis (neurons). In some neurons and endocrine cells, both LDCV and SV exocytosis are found [97-107]. They can be distinguished by morphological appearance of the secretory vesicles and by kinetics of the release [108].

Basic components of the regulated exocytotic apparatus are highly conserved among different secretory cell types [109], allowing to readily demonstrate the initial process of exocytosis in both sympathetic neurons and adrenal chromaffin cells [110, 111]. Despite the differences in the time course, Ca^{2+} dependency, and signal input between LDCV and SV exocytosis, both involve common processes: [1] vesicle recruitment to the plasma membrane, [2] docking of vesicles at the plasma membrane, [3] priming of fusion machinery, and [4] fusion of vesicles with the plasma membrane [110, 111]. The fusion of vesicles is a crucial event in the regulated exocytosis in multicellular organisms, and is tightly controlled to release vesicle contents in response to specific signals, often in a specialized region of the plasma membrane [112]. The final step of the exocytosis process consists in the release of RRP. This release is carried out for the most part by proteins identical or very similar to those functioning at synapses [113]. Although these processes are central to understanding the exocytosis, they are difficult to distinguish by current available methods.

Despite the Ca^{2+} ions being messengers vital to the exocytosis, an increase of the $(Ca^{2+})_c$ is a basic requirement for the release of neurotransmitters from sympathetic neurons, and hormones from adrenal chromaffin cells; this process (exocytosis) involves other intracellular messengers, including IP_3, PKC, diacylglycerol (DAG) and cAMP [114-116]. The exact role of these intracellular messengers in the fine regulation of exocytosis in neurons and neuroendocrine cells remains under investigation [117, 118]. Thus, the knowledge of a precise Ca^{2+} signalling involved in the exocytosis process, and its interaction with other intracellular messengers in the release of neurotransmitters from sympathetic neurons, and hormones from adrenal chromaffin cells, is crucial for the comprehension of autonomic and central neurotransmission in physiological situations, and pathological conditions.

Chapter 3

CA^{2+} SIGNALLING INVOLVED IN THE EXOCYTOSIS OF NEUROENDOCRINE CELLS: BASIC CONCEPTS FOR UNDERSTANDING NEUROLOGICAL AND PSYCHIATRIC DISEASES

A series of experiments initiated 60 years ago using chromaffin cells as cellular models originated the concept of the stimulus-secretion coupling to explain the neurotransmitter release, and hormone secretion. This concept initially derived from the study of cat adrenal gland perfused with ACh performed by Douglas and Rubin in 1960s [63]. The discovery that an increase of the $(Ca^{2+})c$ is a basic requirement for exocytosis in adrenal chromaffin cells was made by Baker and Knight in 1970s [119]. In addition to Ca^{2+}, Holz et al. demonstrated in 1980s that the exocytosis in adrenal chromaffin cells was also dependent of ATP [120].

The most direct demonstration of a relationship between a rise in $(Ca^{2+})c$ and a rapid exocytosis derived from the study performed by Neher and Zucker in 1990s using photo released Ca^{2+}-caged in adrenal chromaffin cells, which revealed the multiple Ca^{2+}-dependent steps of exocytosis [121]. Subsequent studies performed by Neher and Sudhof in 2000s showed that the Ca^{2+}-dependent steps of exocytosis were similar in neurons and neuroendocrine cells [88, 108]. Erwin Neher was awarded with the Nobel Prize in Physiology or Medicine in 1991 for his discoveries concerning the function of single ion channels in cells, and Thomas Sudhof was awarded with the Nobel Prize in Physiology or Medicine in 2013 for his discoveries of the cellular machinery regulating vesicle traffic.

Actually, it is clear the notion that the neurotransmitter release, hormone secretion and a variety of other secretory processes are tightly regulated with exocytotic fusion of secretory vesicles being triggered by a rise in $(Ca^{2+})c$. It is also clear that the *"fight or flight"* response basically depends on the exocytotic release of neurotransmitters from postsynaptic sympathetic neurons, and hormones from adrenal chromaffin cells, triggered by a transient elevation of the $[Ca^{2+}]c$, in response to a stimulation of the nicotinic cholinergic receptors on the surface of these cells by ACh, released from the ending nerves of preganglionic neurons [14, 38, 69, 70, 110, 111]. Although the control of $(Ca^{2+})c$ by these cells is vital to their secretory activity, this control is complex and depends on various cellular elements and processes, which include Ca^{2+} channels, cytosolic Ca^{2+} buffers, the uptake and release of Ca^{2+} from cytoplasmic organelles, such as endoplasmic reticulum (ER), mitochondria (MIT), chromaffin vesicles and the nucleus, and Ca^{2+} extrusion mechanisms [14, 38, 69, 70, 110, 111].

The Ca^{2+} entry into the cytosol of excitable cells is regulated by various types of plasmalemmal Ca^{2+} channels, including VACC, ligand-gated Ca^{2+} and store-operated Ca^{2+} channels [14, 69, 70]. The VACC constitute the most relevant Ca^{2+} entry pathway that triggers the release of hormones from chromaffin cells, and neurotransmitters from sympathetic neurons [14, 38, 69, 70, 110, 111]. This Ca^{2+} influx through VACC promotes a transient elevation of the $(Ca^{2+})_c$, which stimulates a Ca^{2+} release from the ER into the cytosol due to an activation of the ryanodine receptor channel (RyR) [14, 38, 69, 70, 110, 111]. Known as Ca^{2+}-induced Ca^{2+} release (CICR), this mechanism amplifies the Ca^{2+} signals, stimulating the exocytosis in neurons and neuroendocrine cells [14]. The Ca^{2+} release from the ER is also mediated by an activation of an $InsP_3$ receptor channel (IP_3R) by $InsP_3$ generated by an activation of G-protein coupled membrane receptors, such as muscarinic cholinergic receptors [14, 38].

The ER of chromaffin cells behaves as a single thapsigargin-sensitive Ca^{2+} pool that can release Ca^{2+} both via CICR or IP_3R [14]. For example, using bovine chromaffin cells transfected with ER-targeted aequorin for monitoring the ER Ca^{2+} concentration ($(Ca^{2+})_{ER}$), it was shown that a Ca^{2+} entry elicited by a membrane depolarization by ACh triggers a transient Ca^{2+} release from the ER that is highly dependent on $(Ca^{2+})_{ER}$, and sensitized by low caffeine concentrations [14]. In addition, treatment of these cells with a mixture of caffeine, ryanodine and thapsigargin produced severe ER Ca^{2+} depletion of the catecholamine release stimulated by ACh [14]. These findings indicate that ACh elicits a discrete, and more localized, $(Ca^{2+})_c$ elevation, and the contribution of the CICR to the exocytotic response is more visible under conditions of physiological stimulation of the chromaffin cells by cholinergic transmitter [14]. Thus, activation of the CICR during cell depolarization may have functional consequences for the control of the exocytotic process.

Mitochondria (MIT) also have an important role in the control of $(Ca^{2+})_c$ and of exocytosis in neuroendocrine cells, and in neurons. Known as the main energy-producing centers of eukaryotic cells, MIT are capable of accumulating vast amounts of Ca^{2+} in their matrix through their MIT Ca^{2+} uniporter (MU), that uses the driving force of the electrical potential across the MIT membrane [122-124]. The MIT matrix is more negative than the cytosol, with a large transmembrane potential difference (~ −180 mV) that is generated by the respiratory chain or by the ATP hydrolysis [123, 124]. Ca^{2+} accumulated into MIT matrix is released back into the cytosol by electroneutral antiporters that export Ca^{2+} from the matrix by swapping one Ca^{2+} ion for two Na^+ through the MIT Na^+/Ca^{2+} exchanger (mNCX) [14]. During a cell activation, some MIT take up Ca^{2+} from cytosolic Ca^{2+} microdomains (HCMDs) that are created by the opening of nearby VACC [125, 126]. It was shown in rat chromaffin cells that MIT act as rapid and reversible Ca^{2+} buffers during a cell stimulation [127], and in bovine chromaffin cells it was shown that MIT contribute to the clearance of large

Ca^{2+} loads [125, 128], and exhibit surprisingly rapid millimolar Ca^{2+} transients upon a cell stimulation with ACh [129].

The plasma membrane Ca^{2+}-ATPase (PMCA) and Na^+/Ca^{2+} exchanger (NCX) constitute the main transport systems to extrude Ca^{2+} from the intracellular into the extracellular compartment [14]. Both transporters contribute to maintain the long-term Ca^{2+} homeostasis through a well-balanced Ca^{2+} influx and Ca^{2+} efflux activities. The functional expression of these two transporters was first demonstrated using plasma membrane vesicles from the bovine adrenal medulla [130]. The PMCA has a high Ca^{2+} affinity (K_D ~ 0.1 µM) and operates as an electrogenic Ca^{2+}/H^+ exchanger with a 1:1 stoichiometry [131]. The NCX uses the energy provided by the Na^+ gradient to achieve an electrogenic exchange of 3 Na^+ ions for 1 Ca^{2+}.

Under physiological conditions, Na^+ is transported into the cell and Ca^{2+} is extruded from the cytosol [132]. However, when the electrochemical gradient for Na^+ is reversed, such as during membrane depolarization or the opening of gated Na^+ channels, the NCX moves Na^+ out of the cell and Ca^{2+} into the cell [133]. The Ca^{2+} exit mode is referred to as the *forward mode*, and the Ca^{2+} entry mode as the *reverse mode* of the NCX [134]. The NCX1, major isoform of the NCX expressed by bovine chromaffin cells [135, 136], mediates a Na^+-dependent Ca^{2+} influx [137] or a Ca^{2+} export [138] depending on the circumstances. In these cells, NCX1 can favor a Na^+-dependent Ca^{2+} influx [137] or a Ca^{2+} export [138], and participates in the regulation of $(Ca^{2+})c$ and of exocytosis [135-139].

Using adrenal chromaffin cells as cellular models, Garcia and collaborators [14] proposed *"functional Ca^{2+} tetrads"* theory to explain how neuroendocrine cells and neurons shape the Ca^{2+} transients during a cell activation to regulate early and late steps of exocytosis, and the ensuing endocytotic responses. In accordance to this theory, these cells have developed *"functional Ca^{2+} tetrads"* formed by the VACC, cytosolic Ca^{2+} buffers, the ER, and MIT nearby the exocytotic plasmalemmal sites to shape Ca^{2+} gradients and Ca^{2+} microdomains [14]. The *"functional Ca^{2+} tetrads"* (see Figure 3.1) is activated by a direct membrane depolarization or action potentials fired by the interaction of ACh with nicotinic receptors on the surface of chromaffin cells [71]. This event is likely the primary stimulus that induces the $(Ca^{2+})c$ transient, thus triggering the discharge of adrenaline and noradrenaline from chromaffin cells into the circulation, and noradrenaline into the sympathetic synapses [92].

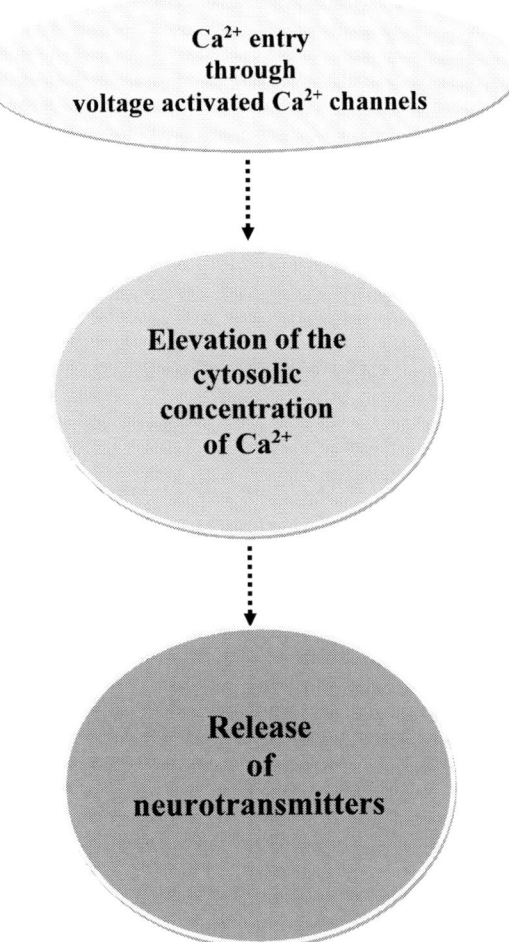

Figure 3.1. The VACC constitute the most relevant Ca^{2+} entry pathway that triggers the release of hormones from chromaffin cells, and neurotransmitters from sympathetic neurons. This Ca^{2+} influx through VACC promotes a transient elevation of the $(Ca^{2+})c$, which stimulates a Ca^{2+} release from the ER into the cytosol due to an activation of the ryanodine receptor channel (RyR).

Ca^{2+} entry through the various subtypes of VACC (L, N, and P/Q) is the primary determinant for the extent and shape of the initial $(Ca^{2+})c$ transient. However, cytosolic Ca^{2+} buffers, Ca^{2+} sequestration or a release from the cytoplasmic organelles, and plasmalemmal Ca^{2+} extrusion have a prominent role in the fine tuning of the Ca^{2+} signal. On the other hand, correct Ca^{2+} signalling is critical to warrant the adaptation of the entire organism to a stress response which determines its survival.

Essential for understanding the Ca^{2+} function in chromaffin cells is the concept that the organelles and cytosolic Ca^{2+} buffer shape $(Ca^{2+})c$ transients at different cell locations, the so-called high-Ca^{2+} microdomains (HCMDs), that do not necessarily crosstalk. Several kinds of these HCMDs have been described in different cell systems and given evocative names, such as sparks, puffs, sparklers and syntillas [140, 141]. Syntillas are brief focal $(Ca^{2+})_c$ transients elicited by a localized ER Ca^{2+} release via RyR channels, first reported in the neurohypophysial terminals at magnocellular neurons [142]. These focal Ca^{2+} transients were later on found in mouse chromaffin cells [143] and, paradoxically, they seem to block the spontaneous exocytosis in these cells [144]. Because CICR is present in bovine chromaffin cells, it could be of interest to investigate whether the Ca^{2+} wave that extends from the subplasmalemmal sites to the inner cytosol following a 100 ms depolarizing pulse, and CICR activation [145], is composed of elementary syntillas. It seems that the presence and functional role for the Ca^{2+} syntillas are seriously questioned, and controversial.

The rates of the Ca^{2+} fluxes between different chromaffin cell compartments have been estimated using more or less direct approaches, and under temperature conditions (i.e., room temperature) that might affect the activity of some Ca^{2+} transporters. Even with these limitations, putting together the estimates of the different fluxes allows for several interesting predictions [125]. For instance, for a 15 μm diameter bovine chromaffin cell, a rate of Ca^{2+} entry of 700 μmol L . cells^{-1} . s^{-1} can be computed from the measured Ca^{2+} inward current [146]. A similar value (400 μmol L. cells^{-1} . s^{-1}) was estimated by measuring $^{45}Ca^{2+}$ uptake into K$^+$ depolarized bovine chromaffin cells [147]. Ca^{2+} entry would be focused at the channels locations, and then diffuses through the surrounding cytosol. Regarding progression of the Ca^{2+} wave generated by Ca^{2+} entry through plasma membrane Ca^{2+} channels, binding to cytosolic Ca^{2+} buffers is a most important determinant. The cytosol of bovine chromaffin cells has a Ca^{2+} binding capacity of ~ 4 mmol/L cells. The cytosolic calcium buffers are scarcely mobile and have a low Ca^{2+} affinity (K_D ~100 µM) with an activity coefficient of ~ 1/40 [128,146]. The two-dimensional diffusion coefficient is ~40 µm^2/s and shows inhomogeneities at the nuclear envelope, and at the plasma membrane [148]. Brief openings of VACC generate HCMDs near the channel mouth that can be detected in Ca^{2+} imaging measurements [149]. These HCMDs can reach concentrations as high as 10 - 100 µM [50, 149]. Because of rapid diffusion of Ca^{2+} towards the surrounding cytosol, the HCMDs are highly restricted in time and space [50, 150]. The presence of mobile Ca^{2+} buffers accelerates diffusion and opposes the development of HCMDs [146, 151-153], for example, at concentrations of 50 µM; fura-2 increases the apparent rate of the Ca^{2+} diffusion four times [146].

Ca^{2+} entering into the cell redistributes among the different cell compartments. The increase of $(Ca^{2+})_c$ activates the sarco-endoplasmic reticulum Ca^{2+}-ATPase (SERCA), and the ER avidly takes up Ca^{2+} from the cytosol. For example, during a stimulation of chromaffin cells from bovine [146] and rat [154], the maximal Ca^{2+} uptake by the ER ranges between 40 and 80 µmol L . cells^{-1} . s^{-1}. At rest, the rate of Ca^{2+} exchange between ER and cytosol at steady state is 2 - 3 µmol L. cells^{-1} . s^{-1}. The net Ca^{2+} influx upon maximal stimulation with caffeine or InsP$_3$-producing agonists is 10 - 20 times faster [145].

Concerning MIT, it is notorious that the Ca^{2+} activity coefficient (free Ca^{2+}/bound Ca^{2+}) in the matrix is very low, in the 1/1000 range [125, 127]. MIT are very effective in the clearing of $(Ca^{2+})_c$ transients, although drastic differences have been reported between bovine and rat chromaffin cells. For instance, in experiments with photo release of caged Ca^{2+} in bovine chromaffin cells, rates of $(Ca^{2+})_{MIT}$ increase as high as 4,800 µmol L. cells^{-1} . s^{-1} were found, and saturating $(Ca^{2+})_c$ at 200 µM [128]. In contrast, MIT uptake rates in rat chromaffin cells are 150 - 300-fold slower, but at $(Ca^{2+})_c$ of only 0.2 - 2 µM [154]. These differences are consistent with dependence of the rate of uptake through the MU on the second power of $(Ca^{2+})_c$ [155-157].

Using MIT-targeted aequorin to specifically monitor $(Ca^{2+})_{MIT}$, it was found that MIT took up about 1,100 µmol L . cells^{-1} . s^{-1} upon maximal stimulation of Ca^{2+} entry into bovine chromaffin cells depolarized with high K$^+$ [115, 125, 129, 156]; this value is comparable with the rate of Ca^{2+} entry through VACC. The maximal rate of Ca^{2+} release from MIT trough the MIT Na$^+$/Ca^{2+} exchanger (mNCX) at 37°C in bovine chromaffin cells is about 800 µmol . cells^{-1} . s^{-1} [115]. Regarding the kinetics of this MIT Ca^{2+} efflux, the dependence on $(Ca^{2+})_{MIT}$ is exponential and the K$_{50}$ approaches 200 µM [125]. Transport through the MU is usually unidirectional (entry); however, when MIT are completely depolarized, the uniporter may allow Ca^{2+} exit from the matrix in a sort of MIT CICR mechanism [156]. In rat chromaffin cells, the joint action of both PMCA and NCX to extrude Ca^{2+} from the cell has been estimated to decrease $(Ca^{2+})_c$ to a maximal rate of 20 µmol L . cells^{-1} . s^{-1} at 27°C [154, 158] and 100 µmol L . cells^{-1} . s^{-1} at 37°C [115,125].

At each moment, the $(Ca^{2+})_c$ is defined by the rate of Ca^{2+} redistribution into chromaffin cell compartments, which in turn depends on fluxes between the extracellular medium, the cytosol, cytosolic Ca^{2+} buffers and organelles. At rest, a steady state with Ca^{2+} exchange rates below 10 µmol L . cells^{-1} . s^{-1}, and $(Ca^{2+})_c$ near 0.1 µM is established; $(Ca^{2+})_{MIT}$ is similar to $(Ca^{2+})_c$ while $(Ca^{2+})_{ER}$ is much higher, reaching 500 – 1,000 µM. Consequently, there are enormous electrochemical gradients favoring Ca^{2+} diffusion into the cytosol from both the ER and the extracellular medium, where the Ca^{2+} concentration is above 1 mM.

At low-frequency stimulation with action potentials, the rate of Ca^{2+} diffusion through the cytosol and binding by the endogenous Ca^{2+} buffers are the main determinants of the $(Ca^{2+})c$ signal [50, 150]. Under these conditions, global $(Ca^{2+})c$ goes up to about 1 µM, and then the Ca^{2+} clearance is primarily achieved through the high-affinity Ca^{2+}-ATPase and through SERCA. Upon strong stimulation (high-frequency action potentials or prolonged depolarization), global $(Ca^{2+})c$ may approach 10 µM, a concentration high enough to activate Ca^{2+} uptake through the MU. Under these conditions, most of the Ca^{2+} that enters into the chromaffin cells is taken up by MIT [115, 125, 129, 154, 158]. For example, MIT targeted aequorin revealed that 90% of the Ca^{2+} that enters into a bovine chromaffin cell stimulated with a 10-s K^+ pulse is taken up by MIT. Later, when the stimulation ceases, the Ca^{2+} accumulated into the MIT is released back into the cytosol during a period of seconds or even minutes [125]. The Ca^{2+} accumulated into the MIT stimulates respiration until Ca^{2+} extrusion from the MIT matrix is completed [125]. It can be speculated that the extra energy provided in this way may be used for clearing the Ca^{2+} load and restoring the Ca^{2+} homeostasis after the activity period.

In bovine chromaffin cells, the opening of VACC generates HCMDs of about 0.3 μm of diameter and 10 μM of $(Ca^{2+})_c$ [149, 159-161]. Building of HCMDs may be favored by a colocalization of VACC clusters and chromaffin vesicles [162-164]. Evanescent microscopy has shown fast ($t_{1/2}$ ~100 ms) and localized [~ 350 nm] HCMDs beneath the plasma membrane of stimulated chromaffin cells [165]. These HCMDs selectively trigger the release of vesicles docked within 300 nm, indicating that some vesicles are docked but not primed. It is interesting that HCMDs reduce the distance between the docked vesicles and Ca^{2+} entry sites, suggesting a role for the stimulation-dependent facilitation of exocytosis in chromaffin cells [164,165].

MIT located nearby VACC at subplasmalemmal sites can sense HCMDs during a physiological stimulation [125,129,154,158]. Through measurements of aequorin consumption upon repeated stimulation of bovine chromaffin cells, the cumulative history of Ca^{2+} uptake may be traced. Using this approach, two pools of MIT with different subcellular distribution were evidenced. Pool M1, located nearby exocytotic sites, accumulates (Ca2+)c at a rate of 2,000 μmol L . cells^{-1} . s^{-1}, while pool M2 located at inner cytosolic areas takes up Ca^{2+} at a much lower rate, 12 μmol L. cells^{-1} . s^{-1} [125, 129]. These rates are reached at concentrations of 20 and 2 μM of $(Ca^{2+})_c$ respectively, which are coincident with the concentrations reached at subplasmalemmal sites, and the cell core during a cell stimulation. The M1 pool would tune the MIT function to match the local energy needed for the exocytosis and Ca^{2+} redistribution, whereas the M2 pool, located at the bulk cytosol, could serve to redistribute the Ca^{2+} and canalize it towards inner cytosolic regions to serve other cell functions, i.e., transport of new secretory vesicles into plasmalemmal exocytotic sites.

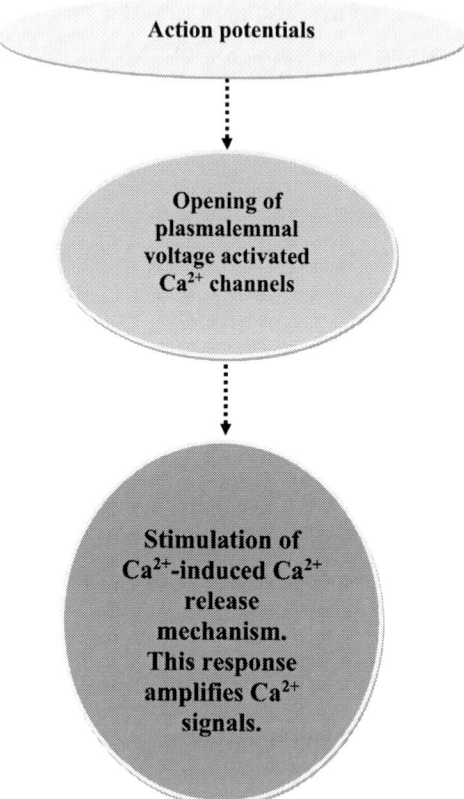

Figure 3.2 "Functional tetrad hypothesis" to explain the cellular Ca^{2+} homeostasis involved in exocytosis in the adrenal chromaffin cells. Propagation of fire action potentials in chromaffin cells promotes the opening of plasmalemmal VACC (L, N and P/Q- types), producing a transient elevation of $(Ca^{2+})_c$. This response stimulates Ca^{2+}-induced Ca^{2+} release (CICR) mechanism from the ER due to an activation by Ca^{2+} of Ca^{2+}-channels controlled by the ryanodine receptors (RyR). This response amplifies $(Ca^{2+})_c$, and in turn, stimulating exocytosis of secretory vesicles rich in catecholamines. Ca^{2+} sequestration into, and Ca^{2+} release from, the cytoplasmic organelles, such as ER and MIT participate of regulation of $(Ca^{2+})_c$. This functional tetrad controls pre-exocytotic and exocytotic steps in the process of regulating the secretory response in neuroendocrine cells.

ER Ca^{2+} fluxes could also contribute to the regulation of HCMDs formed during cell stimulation. For instance, under K^+-depolarization of bovine chromaffin cells transfected with ER-targeted aequorin, reductions of 60 - 100 µM $(Ca^{2+})_{ER}$ are observed (about 10 - 15% of the total ER Ca^{2+} content) [145], suggesting a CICR. Although the decrease of $(Ca^{2+})_{ER}$ may see quite small, it could correspond to a large release at certain subcellular ER locations compensated by strong uptake in others. CICR sites seem to co-localize with the plasmalemmal VACC and the M1 MIT pool. Thus, the complex functional tetrads including VACC, cytosolic Ca^{2+} buffers, the MU and the RyR are essential for the efficacious regulation of the adequate local $(Ca^{2+})_c$ transients to control the rate and extent of exocytotic release of neurotransmitter and hormones. A model of a functional tetrad involved in the exocytosis of hormone from adrenal chromaffin cells adapted from Garcia and collaborators [14] is shown in Figure 3.2.

Chromaffin cells have been thoroughly used as models to study the relationship between Ca^{2+} entry, cytosolic Ca^{2+} signals, exocytosis and endocytosis, using patch-clamp and amperometric techniques. Cells have been stimulated with single depolarizing pulses (DPs), DP trains and with simulated AP waveforms. These approaches have provided useful information, but we have no data on APs generated by pulsatile secretory quanta of ACh, trying to mimic the intermittent and repetitive splanchnic nerve discharge of the neurotransmitter. Ultrashort pulses of a high ACh concentration (1000 µM) cause a single AP followed by a prolonged depolarization. It could be interesting trying to correlate these "patterns of splanchnic nerve discharge" with Ca^{2+} signals and the exocytosis. This, together with the use of adrenal slices and transmural electrical stimulation of splanchnic nerves, will provide new physiologically sound data on the regulation of the adrenal medullary secretion.

The chromaffin cell has also been used as a model to characterize releasable components present in the secretory granules, and to understand the cellular mechanisms involved in the catecholamine release. The development of high resolution methodologies to detect catecholamines released from the chromaffin cells has been decisive to understand the exocytosis in neuroendocrine cells and neurons. For instance, the detection of adrenaline and noradrenaline from bovine adrenal chromaffin cells, using amperometry techniques with carbon fiber microelectrode, allows measure in real time of a single vesicle containing catecholamines. In addition, this approach allows the detailed investigation of the presynaptic response at the single cell level with a single vesicle resolution, including the regulation of signalling pathways [166]. Characterization of the regulated exocytosis in chromaffin cells not only provides fundamental knowledge of neurosecretion, but is also of importance, as these cells are used for therapeutic purposes. An illustration of high resolution amperometric technique using carbon fiber microelectrode for the study of catecholamine exocytosis in adrenal chromaffin is shown in Figure 3.2. Thus, the knowledge of the precise Ca^{2+} signalling involved in the exocytosis process, and its interaction with other intracellular messengers, like cAMP, in the release of neurotransmitters from sympathetic neurons, and hormones from adrenal chromaffin cells, is crucial for the comprehension of autonomic and central neurotransmission in physiological situations, and in pathological conditions.

Chapter 4

ROLE OF cAMP IN THE EXOCYTOSIS OF THE NEUROENDOCRINE CELLS: FUNDAMENTAL CONCEPTS FOR STUDYING NEUROLOGICAL AND PSYCHIATRIC DISEASES

Some studies showed that cAMP is involved in the fine regulation of exocytosis from different cell types of vertebrates, including sympathetic [80, 81] and parasympathetic ganglion neurons [82], and yet increases the catecholamines secretion from adrenal chromaffin cells [41, 43, 83, 84]. Although the cellular, and molecular, mechanisms involved in these regulatory actions of cAMP on the exocytosis of neurotransmitter and hormones are unclear, the evidences suggest that this intracellular messenger can thus participate in the fine regulation of exocytosis due to its modulatory action on the intracellular Ca^{2+} signals.

An elevation of the $(Ca^{2+})_c$ is not only involved in the late steps of exocytosis but is also involved in the earlier steps. Thus, the filling of the RRP, measured as a recovery from depletion, was enhanced by a mild elevation of the $(Ca^{2+})_c$ induced either by a moderate depolarization or by histamine (159, 167). Heinemann et al. [168] incorporated the Ca^{2+}-

dependent vesicle supply to the RRP, and observed that the model adequately explained the depression and augmentation of the exocytosis.

Bergantin et al (2013) [6] proposed that the increase of cAMP intracellular levels induces a Ca^{2+} release from the ER, increasing the number of vesicles near the plasmalemma, and thus facilitating the neurotransmitter release from sympathetic nerves. This process frees vesicles from the cytoskeletal barrier and allows them to translocate into the active secretory sites under the plasmalemma. This effect of cAMP enhancers appears to be mediated by the PKA stimulation. However, the involvement of PKA deserves further experimental attention. Several intracellular messengers participate in the Ca^{2+}-triggered exocytosis [114-116]. Several studies showed that cAMP participates in the exocytosis regulation in a variety of secretory cells, including in neurons and in neuroendocrine cells [64, 115, 169-178]. In neurons, cAMP has been shown to induce a long-term potentiation (LTP) [179-181] by increasing the neurotransmitter release at mossy fiber synapses in the hippocampus of cerebrum [182, 183], and at parallel fiber-Purkinje neuron synapses in the cerebellum [184, 185]. cAMP increases the transmitter release at many synapses in the vertebrate peripheral ganglia and in the invertebrate nervous systems, including in sympathetic [80, 81, 186] and parasympathetic ganglion neurons [82], in neuromuscular junctions of *crayfish* [187], in central synapses of *Aplysia* [188-192], and in neuromuscular junctions of *Drosophila melanogaster [Drosophila]*[193] .

In endocrine cells, cAMP regulates the release of various hormones, including the pancreatic hormones such as insulin from pancreatic β-cells [194-198], glucagon from pancreatic β-cells [199, 200], pituitary hormones such as adrenocorticotropin (ACTH) from pituitary corticotropes [201-203], catecholamines from adrenal chromaffin cells [41, 43, 83, 84] and a myriad of other cellular processes [204, 205].

In exocrine parotid acinar cells, cAMP, rather than Ca^{2+}, is the primary signal in the amylase release [170, 206]. PKA has been thought to be the major target of cAMP in cAMP-regulated exocytosis in multicellular organisms. However, cAMP is now known to have other targets as well, including the cyclic nucleotide-gated (CNG) channels [207], the hyperpolarization-activated cyclic nucleotide-gated (HCN) channels [208] and the cAMP-specific guanine nucleotide exchange factors (cAMP-GEF)/exchange proteins directly activated by cAMP (Epac) (here after cAMP-GEF/Epac) [209, 210]. Although the PKA-dependent mechanisms of regulation, and modulation, of the exocytosis by cAMP have been studied extensively [64, 115, 169-178], the PKA-independent mechanisms are currently being unveiled. The cAMP-regulated exocytosis in adrenal chromaffin cells is shown in Figure 4.1. In this book, we also discussed how the interaction between the intracellular signalling pathways mediated by Ca^{2+} and cAMP can finely regulate the exocytosis in the sympathetic neurons and adrenal chromaffin cells, and yet how this interaction can attenuate the neuronal death in the neurodegenerative diseases resulted from a cytosolic Ca^{2+} excess. The hypothesis for a functional interaction between the intracellular signalling pathways mediated by Ca^{2+} or cAMP has been extensively studied in a myriad cell and tissue systems; this interaction is the key of the "calcium paradox" concept. Generally, this interaction results in synergistic effects on cell functions [211-213] and occurs at the level of AC or PDE. In general, AC5 and AC6 isoforms are inhibited by a physiological increase of $(Ca^{2+})c$ [212-214], as indicated in Figure 4.1. Figure 4.1 illustrates that when excitable cells are stimulated by a membrane depolarization, a Ca^{2+} influx mediated mainly by the L-type VACC promotes an increase of $(Ca^{2+})c$, which inhibits the AC activity, and in turn reduces the intracellular cAMP levels, resulting in a reduction of cellular responses mediated by the cAMP signalling pathways [212, 214]. Recent data suggest that the compartmentalization of AC may also cause functional compartmentalization and $(cAMP)_c$ oscillations. The more precise and specific compartmentalization takes place within several AC in proximity to the VACC. Thus, in excitable cells, Ca^{2+}-regulated AC are modulated by a Ca^{2+} entry through the VACC [215]. Not surprisingly, the form of regulation reported in most studies is that in which AC are regulated by a Ca^{2+} influx through the VACC.

Calcium also regulates the activity of several PDE, an issue that nevertheless has been studied to a lesser extent [216]. The specific function of the PDE, and their interaction with Ca^{2+}, likely contribute to the generation of cAMP microdomains. This is described in detail in a recent study that examined the response of two PDE1 isoforms to a Ca^{2+} influx through store-operated Ca^{2+} channels (SOCCs) [217]. Such interaction has also been demonstrated in pancreatic acini [218], in parotid acini [31], in blowfly salivary glands [34], in hepatocytes [32], in airway epithelial cells [33], in cardiac myocytes [219], in skeletal myocytes [220], and in neurons [221]. Then, this functional Ca^{2+}/cAMP interaction importantly participates in the regulation of cellular response in various cell types. Studies performed by Bergantin et al. [6] indicated that this interaction is involved in the exocytosis of neuroendocrine cells (see Figure 4.1).

The Ca^{2+}/cAMP interaction has particularly been extensively studied at the Ca^{2+} channels of the ER [222-224]. But, is this interaction operational and functionally relevant in normal neuroendocrine cells? Correlated molecular and pharmacological analysis showed that in rat adenohypophyseal corticotrope cells, Ca^{2+} mobilized from the ryanodine-sensitive ER Ca^{2+} stores (via RyR channels) suppressed the cAMP synthesis induced by physiological concentrations of corticotropin releasing-factor (CRF); and the plausible targets for Ca^{2+} are AC9 cells [213]. Activation of RyR channels, and the consequent release of Ca^{2+} into the cytoplasm, may be regulated by cAMP through the RyR-associated kinase/phosphatase complexes, the dynamics of which are bound to vary with the type of system remains under investigation [213]. Phosphorylation of the RyR by PKA, and also IP_3R at submaximal IP_3 concentrations, may increase the open probability of the ER Ca^{2+} stores, amplifying the CICR mechanism and cellular responses [213] (Figure 4.1).

In addition to cAMP, many studies have shown that the different proteins involved in the intracellular signalling are also targets for Ca^{2+}. For example, it was shown that the activation of PKC by phorbol 12-myristate 13-acetate (PMA) potentiates the responses to different secretagogues [225-229]. PMA does not induce the exocytosis by itself but causes the disruption of the cortical F-actin network, a barrier that blocks the vesicle movement towards the plasma membrane [230-232] and doubles the number of vesicles at 50 nm below the plasmalemma, as well as the secretion response [233]. This effect of PMA was blocked by PKC inhibitors, confirming the involvement of PKC [233, 234]. The effect of PMA was mimicked by K$^+$ and nicotine, which stimulate a Ca^{2+} entry and the exocytosis. Thus, Ca^{2+} activates a PKC-mediated phosphorylation step that causes the disruption of the cortical actin network. This process frees vesicles from the cytoskeletal barrier and allows them to translocate into active secretory sites under the plasmalemma.

Gillis et al. [235] confirmed that the PMA activates PKC, and then enhances the release. PMA augments the size of the RRP, without changing the probability of release from DVP. This conclusion was supported by the fact that PMA selectively increased the amplitude of the exocytotic burst induced by photo released Ca^{2+}, but it did not modify the kinetics of the secretory response. Smith et al. [236] showed that the PKC activation doubled the RRP by doubling the rate constant for vesicle supply. In addition, reducing the basal (Ca^{2+})$_c$ reduced the RRP, while increasing (Ca^{2+})$_c$ raised the RRP, showing a direct relationship between (Ca^{2+})$_c$ and the release of secretory response. The authors showed that the increase of RRP may be attributed, at a moderate (Ca^{2+})$_c$, to the direct action of Ca^{2+} on the transition rate; however, indirect effects through PKC may contribute to the large effects of a 500 nM basal (Ca^{2+})$_c$. Later experiments using trains of depolarizing stimuli reached the same conclusion [237]. Again, a direct Ca^{2+}-dependent action and an indirect, long-lasting effect through PKC, were distinguished. Vitale et al. [233] suggested that the PKC promotes the recruitment and docking of vesicles, while those of Gillis et al. [235], Smith et al. [236] and Smith [237] indicate a stimulatory action of Ca^{2+} and PKC on priming, a post docking action. It is also intriguing that the Munc-13, a protein involved in the exocytosis, shows a PMA-dependent but PKC-independent activity [238]. On the other hand, Munc-18 phosphorylation in response to PMA treatment of chromaffin cells provides another mechanism for the control of exocytosis in the secretory cells [239]. Furthermore, a PKC-induced phosphorylation of SNAP-25 plays a role in the vesicle recruitment [240].

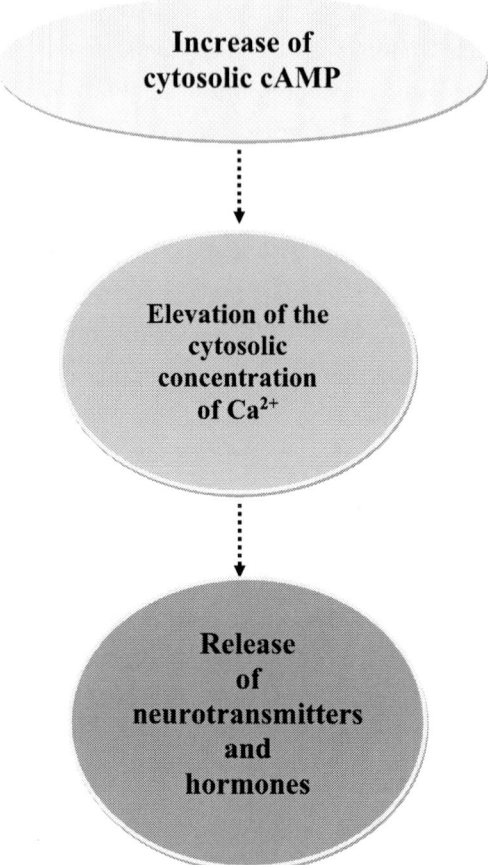

Figure 4.1. cAMP regulates the release of various hormones. The pancreatic hormones such as insulin from pancreatic β-cells, glucagon from pancreatic β-cells, pituitary hormones such as adrenocorticotropin [ACTH] from pituitary corticotropes, catecholamines from adrenal chromaffin cells and a myriad of other cellular processes [204,205] are regulated by cAMP.

In addition to the PKC, other proteins are also targets for Ca^{2+}. Thus, synaptotagmin, which has been proposed as the final Ca^{2+} sensor to trigger the secretory response [241] has been identified in chromaffin cells [242, 243]. Nevertheless, Ca^{2+}-dependent activator protein for the secretion (CAPS) is critical to trigger the exocytosis [244] as by other Ca^{2+} binding proteins. Previous studies of our lab [6] showed that the $(cAMP)_c$ enhancers (Rolipram, IBMX and Forskolin) do not induce a secretory response by themselves, but facilitate the neurotransmission in the electrically-stimulated vas deferens by potentiating the neurotransmitters release from postganglionic sympathetic nerves. Thus, the dysregulation of this mechanism could lead to serious pathological consequences, such as cardiovascular dysfunctions, or could be a novel target for neurological and psychiatric disorders.

Chapter 5

NOVEL CONCEPTS FROM THE CA^{2+}/CAMP INTERACTION: IMPACT IN NEUROLOGICAL AND PSYCHIATRIC DISEASES

Neurological and psychiatric disorders have been considered a severe global illness, becoming more and more common each decade [245]. Because of their devastating symptoms, they have been considered as a leading cause of disability all over the world [245, 246]. Neurological disorders which result from neurodegeneration (neurodegenerative diseases) commonly begin years before a clinical diagnosis can be consistently made (asymptomatic/slightly symptomatic patients), for example Alzheimer's and Parkinson's diseases [247]. The early diagnostic phase of these diseases offers an opportunity for therapies, for example: those aimed to interrupt or preventing the progression of these diseases, and their many complications and side effects, could be of more benefit. However, no such efficient therapies are available at the present moment [247]. Thus, revealing the mechanisms of neurodegeneration from the earliest stages could lead to the development of new interventions, whose therapeutic potential will need to be assessed in adequately designed clinical trials. Advances in the understanding of this early phase of neurodegenerative diseases will lead to the identification of biomarkers of neurodegeneration, and its progression. These biomarkers will help to identify the ideal population to be included, and the most appropriate outcomes to be assessed in clinical trials of medicines. Thus, in this book we discuss novel strategies to treat neurological and psychiatric disorders, throughout our recent discovery entitled the *"calcium paradox"* phenomenon due to the Ca^{2+}/cAMP interaction [6, 14, 15].

5.1. Current Therapies to Treat Neurological and Psychiatric Diseases

Here we discuss the current and novel therapies to treat neurological and psychiatric disorders, including Alzheimer's (AD), Parkinson's (PD) and Huntington's diseases, and depression, spinal muscular atrophy, amyotrophic lateral sclerosis and vascular dementia.

5.1.1 Alzheimer's Disease

Neuritic plaques represent the pathological status of Alzheimer's disease, and are respectively related to the accumulation of the β-amyloid peptide (Aβ) in the brain tissues [248]. According to the amyloid hypothesis, the overproduction of Aβ is a consequence of the disruption of homeostatic processes that regulate the proteolytic cleavage of the amyloid precursor protein (APP). Genetic and age-related factors could contribute to a metabolic change, favoring the amyloidogenic processing of APP in detriment of the physiological secretory pathway [248]. The neurotoxic potential of the Aβ results from its biochemical properties that favor an aggregation. These processes, along with a reduction of Aβ clearance from the brain, lead to the extracellular accumulation of Aβ, and the subsequent activation of neurotoxic cascades that ultimately lead to cytoskeletal changes, neuronal dysfunction and cellular death. Intracerebral amyloidosis development in Alzheimer's disease patients is in an age-dependent manner, but recent evidences indicate that it may be observed in some subjects as early as in the third or fourth decades of life, with an increasing magnitude in late middle age, and highest estimates in old age [245, 248]. The relevance of the early diagnosis of Alzheimer's disease relies on the hypothesis that the pharmacological interventions with disease-modifying compounds are more likely to produce clinically relevant benefits if started early enough in the continuum towards dementia. Therapies targeting the modification of amyloid-related cascades may be viewed as promising strategies to attenuate, or even to prevent dementia [245]. Therefore, the cumulative knowledge on the pathogenesis of Alzheimer's disease derived from the basic science models will hopefully be translated into a clinical practice in the forthcoming years. Other targets relevant to Alzheimer's disease have also been considered in the last years for producing multitarget compounds [249].

In addition to what has been discussed above, acetylcholinesterase (AChE) is another important target to treat the pathogenesis of Alzheimer's disease (cholinergic dysfunction hypothesis). Considering the current hypothesis of an accumulation of the Aβ in Alzheimer's disease, this relies in the reduction of ACh release in the central cholinergic nervous system involved in the cognitive function. Thus, the inhibition of ACh degradation by AChE is a potential target to treat Alzheimer's disease [249]. Deleterious excess of Ca^{2+} influx is also another component seen in aging and in neurodegenerative diseases [250]. Thus, hybrid compounds having the moieties of tacrine, a potent inhibitor of brain and peripheral AChE, and nimodipine, a blocker of L-type CCB have been synthetized [251]. In addition, galantamine, a mild AChE inhibitor and an allosteric ligand of nicotinic receptors has been used to improve the cognition and behavior in patients with Alzheimer's disease. Finally, the N-methyl-D-aspartate (NMDA) receptor antagonist (memantine) has also been proposed to treat this disease.

Besides the current medicines available nowadays in clinics, whose efficacy for treating this disease is limited (Table 5.1), new insights for more efficient pharmacological treatments of Alzheimer's disease are clearly needed.

Table 5.1. List of main medicines for current therapy to treat Alzheimer's disease, including comparison of drugs (efficacy) for treating symptoms

Main medicines to treat Alzheimer's disease and their mechanism of action
Donepezil – AChE inhibitor
Galantamine – mild AChE inhibitor/ligand of nicotinic receptors
Memantine – NMDA receptor antagonist
Rivastigmine – AChE inhibitor
Tacrine – hybrid compound
Efficacy

"There are considerable evidences that the following medicines have modest effects on alleviating symptoms, treating behavioral issues, and improving function in patients with Alzheimer's disease: donepezil, galantamine, rivastigmine, tacrine and memantine. Limited evidences exist on how other medicines compare to these mentioned; there are diverse results for donepezil vs. galantamine. Limited evidences for donepezil vs. rivastigmine suggest only slight differences."

Adapted from "Comparing Alzheimer's Drugs"; https://www.ncbi.nlm.nih.gov/pubmed health/PMH0004911.

5.1.2. Parkinson's Disease

Dopamine loss in the substantia nigra, which results from the reduction of dopamine release in the striatal dopaminergic neurons due to a neuronal death, outcomes in the recognizable core signs of asymmetrical bradykinesia and hypokinesia (slowness and reduced amplitude of movement), muscle rigidity (stiffness) and rest tremor, consequences from modifying the motor control. Rest tremor, prominent asymmetry and a good response to levodopa are the features that most accurately predict the Parkinson's pathology [247]. The tremor-dominant form of Parkinson's tends to run a more benign course than the typical Parkinson's. Early falls or autonomic symptoms, and a response to Parkinson's medicines should raise evidences about the diagnosis [247]. Medication-induced parkinsonism due to commonly prescribed dopamine-blocking medications, such as antipsychotics (e.g., haloperidol, risperidone) and antiemetics (e.g., metoclopramide, prochlorperazine) should be excluded in Parkinson's patients. Functional imaging of the dopaminergic system using a cerebral single photon emission computed tomography, or a positron emission tomography, can be useful in the diagnosis of early Parkinson's. Positron emission tomography studies examining the rate of the decline in dopamine-producing cells suggest that humans have already lost 50%–70% of their nigral neurons, before they develop the motor symptoms, and it has been estimated that the duration of this "pre symptomatic" phase is about 5 years [247]. Early diagnoses will become a critical issue if effective neuroprotective drugs become available. In fact, increasing dopamine, mainly by Levodopa combined with a dopa-decarboxylase inhibitor remains the most potent drug therapy for reversing the motor impairment. A higher maintenance dose of Levodopa (e.g., 200 mg three times daily compared with an initial dose of 100 mg three times daily) provides slightly greater benefit for reducing the motor symptoms, but at the cost of earlier wearing-off the symptoms and dyskinesias [247]. The combination of novel concepts may lead to advances in the Parkinson's research with the promise of finding compounds that are both effective, and fast-acting, including in patients who have tried other therapies with limited success (Table 5.2). In conclusion, new visions for more efficient pharmacological treatments of Parkinson's disease are clearly needed.

Table 5.2. List of main medicines for current therapy to treat Parkinson's disease, including comparison of drugs (efficacy) for treating symptoms

Main medicines to treat Parkinson's disease (PD) and their mechanism of action
Levodopa (LD) – DOPA decarboxylase enzyme substrate
Bromocriptine (BR) – dopamine receptors agonist
Efficacy

"The data revealed no evidence to support the use of early BR/LD combination therapy as a strategy to prevent, or delay the onset of motor complications in the treatment of PD."

Extracted from "Bromocriptine/levodopa combined versus levodopa alone for early Parkinson's disease"; https://www.ncbi.nlm.nih.gov/pubmedhealth/PMH0012203/.

5.1.3. Depression

Depression is an incapacitating psychiatric condition that causes a significant problem on individuals, and on society, by affecting their mood. There is still a lack of a clear understanding of the neuropathological changes associated with this illness, and the efficacy of the antidepressants is still far from the best [246]. Research into antidepressant therapies has derived from observations in human trials and animal models after the first monoaminergic hypothesis emerged (about six decades ago). Nonetheless, the monoamine hypothesis of depression continues to dominate the field and clinical trials, which postulates that an imbalance in monoaminergic neurotransmission is causally related to the clinical features of depression [246]. Antidepressants influence serotonin whose main goal consist of raising serotonin concentrations, thereby increasing the serotonergic transmission at the level of the synapse, for example by inhibiting the serotonin transporter. However, the neuronal transporter serotonin system is multifaceted. Different serotonin receptor subtypes turn the serotonergic system into a complex neurochemical arrangement that influences diverse neurotransmitters in various brain regions. Classical antidepressants, as well as other psychopharmacological agents have various crucial effects on the serotonin receptors. Researchers aim to provide a useful characterization of serotonin receptor subtypes in the treatment of depression. Clarifying the mode of action, and the interplay of serotonin receptors with pharmacological agents should help to elucidate the antidepressant mechanisms and the typical side effects to provide a better understanding. In addition, clinical medicine featured the novel antidepressants vortioxetine, vilazodone and milnacipran/levomilnacipran with regard to their serotonin receptor targets such as the 5-HT1A, 5-HT3 and 5-HT7, which may account for their specific effects on certain symptoms of depression as well as characteristic side-effects profile [246].

In addition to the monoamine hypothesis of depression, glutamatergic modulators, such as ketamine also have become the forefront of antidepressant exploration, especially for the treatment-resistant depression and suicidal ideation [246]. The glutamatergic hypothesis of depression is not novel, however other NMDA receptor modulators do not seem to share the rapid and sustained effects of ketamine, suggesting that a unique combination of intracellular targets might be involved in its effect. Interestingly, inflammation can impact the glutamatergic system enhancing the excitotoxicity and decreasing the neuroplasticity. The points of convergence between the inflammatory and the glutamatergic hypotheses of depression are not completely established, especially regarding the effects of fast-acting antidepressants [246].

Table 5.3. List of main medicines for current therapy to treat depression, including comparison of drugs (efficacy) for treating symptoms

Main medicines to treat Depression and their mechanism of action
Bupropion – reuptake inhibitor of the noradrenaline/dopamine transporter
Citalopram - reuptake inhibitor of the serotonin transporter
Desvenlafaxine - reuptake inhibitor of the noradrenaline/serotonin transporter
Duloxetine - reuptake inhibitor of the noradrenaline/serotonin transporter
Escitalopram - reuptake inhibitor of the serotonin transporter
Fluoxetine - reuptake inhibitor of the serotonin transporter
Fluvoxamine - reuptake inhibitor of the serotonin transporter
Mirtazapine – atypical antidepressant
Nefazodone – 5-HT2A receptor antagonist
Paroxetine - reuptake inhibitor of the serotonin transporter
Sertraline - reuptake inhibitor of the serotonin transporter
Venlafaxine - reuptake inhibitor of the noradrenaline/serotonin transporter
Efficacy

"In general, all of the newer antidepressants are similarly effective in treating major depressive disorder in adults. Although there are some differences in efficacy, the differences are unimportant, and unlikely to be clinically relevant.

For major depressive disorder in children, the strength of the comparative evidences is poor. Compared to placebo, only fluoxetine and escitalopram appear to have some advantage, and may outweigh the risks of treatment, such as the increased risk of suicidal thoughts. Evidence is also partial to how newer antidepressants compare in other depressive disorders, such as dysthymic disorder, subsyndromal depression, and seasonal affective disorder."

Adapted from "Comparing Antidepressants"; https://www.ncbi.nlm.nih.gov/books/ NBK45574

The combination of novel ideas added to the developments on the discoveries may lead to advances in the antidepressant research with the promise of finding compounds that are both effective, and fast-acting, including patients who have used classical therapies (Table 5.3) with limited success. In conclusion, new visions for more efficient pharmacological treatments of depression are clearly needed.

5.1.4. Amyotrophic Lateral Sclerosis (ALS)

Described in 1874 by Jean-Martin Charcot, amyotrophic lateral sclerosis (ALS) is a devastating neurological disease characterized by a progressive muscular paralysis, reflecting a selective degeneration of the motor neurons in the primary motor cortex, brainstem and spinal cord [252]. "Amyotrophy" refers to the atrophy of the skeletal muscle fibers, which are denervated as their corresponding anterior horn cells degenerate, leading into muscle weakness; and "Lateral sclerosis" refers to hardening of the anterior and lateral corticospinal tracts as motor neurons in these areas degenerate, and are replaced by gliosis [253]. ALS is also regarded as a multisystem degeneration with various other signs such as cognitive impairment (sometimes frontotemporal dementia), extrapyramidal features, postural abnormalities, and even small fiber neuropathy, and a mild oculomotor disturbance [252].

ALS is a neurodegenerative disorder that affects both upper (UMN) and lower (LMN) motor neurons. Muscle paralysis is progressive and leads into death due to a respiratory failure within 2–5 years [252]. The incidence of ALS is about 2 per 100,000 persons/years, and its prevalence is about 5 per 100,000 persons. ALS can affect people at any age, but the peak age of onset is 55 to 70 years, with a male predominance (male: female ratio of about 3:2) [254].

The causes of ALS are only partly known, but they include some environmental risk factors as well as several genes that have been identified as harboring a disease-associated variation [252, 255]. Understanding what causes ALS, or what influences against survival, is crucial for the development of effective treatments. Significant advances have been made in understanding the genetic and the environmental components of the disease. In accordance with the Amyotrophic Lateral Sclerosis Online Genetics Database (ALSoD), there are more than 25 genes in which an association with ALS has been replicated, with the rate of gene discovery doubling every 4 years. Most ALS cases are sporadic, but 5–10% of cases are familial, and of these 20% have a mutation of the *SOD1* gene, and about 2–5% have mutations of the *TARDBP* (*TDP-43*) gene. Two percent of apparently sporadic patients have *SOD1* mutations, and *TARDBP* mutations also occur in sporadic cases. There is mixed evidence for the involvement of chemicals, such as heavy metals, ambient aromatic hydrocarbons, pesticides, and cyanotoxins [256-260].

Although the causes of ALS are not fully understood, some evidences suggest that the loss of motor function results from the motor neurons death determined by an imbalance of the intracellular Ca^{2+} homeostasis that causes a cytosolic Ca^{2+} overload [261, 262]. The cytosolic Ca^{2+} overload is also involved in the dysregulation of the glutamatergic signalling and alterations in the neuronal toxicity in ALS [263]. This glutamatergic excitotoxic hypothesis has given rise to an extremely active research field aimed at developing neuroprotective drugs for blocking the excitotoxic process, such as riluzole [263]. Riluzole is the only medication that has proved a modest effect in the survival of ALS patients. Oral administration of riluzole (100 mg daily) improves the 1-year survival by 15% and prolongs survival by 3 months (after 18 months of treatment), with a clear dose response [263]. Long-term use of riluzole was associated with a better prognosis for ALS patients, whereas short-term use had little effect on survival [263]. Then, other neuroprotective pharmacological strategies have been evaluated.

It is well recognized that the interaction between the intracellular signalling pathways mediated by Ca^{2+} and cAMP (Ca^{2+}/cAMP signalling interaction) plays a key role in several cellular processes of mammalians, including in neurotransmission and in neuronal death [6, 14, 15, 264-290]. Our previous studies have indicated that the pharmacological modulation of the Ca^{2+}/cAMP signalling interaction by the combined use of the Ca^{2+} channel blockers (CCBs) and drugs that increment the intracellular concentration of cAMP (cAMP-enhancer compounds) can increase the neurotransmission and can stimulate a neuroprotective response in the neurodegenerative diseases. Then, the pharmacological modulation of the Ca^{2+}/cAMP signalling interaction could open a new avenue for the drug development more effective and safer for treating the neurodegenerative diseases, including ALS. In this book, we discuss the perspectives of the pharmacological modulation of the Ca^{2+}/cAMP signalling interaction as a new therapeutic strategy for ALS, and other neurodegenerative diseases.

5.1.5. Huntington's Disease (HD)

Described in 1872 by American physician George Huntington, the Huntington's disease (HD), also known as Huntington's chorea, is an inherited human neurodegenerative disorder fully penetrant, progressive and fatal [291]. The most characteristic initial physical symptoms are jerky, random, and uncontrollable movements called chorea [291]. The earliest symptoms are often subtle problems with mood or cognitive abilities, and memory deficits tend to appear due to the disease progresses [291]. A general lack of coordination and an unsteady gait often follow [291]. As the disease advances, uncoordinated body movements become more apparent, and cognitive abilities generally decline into dementia [291, 292]. Especially affected are executive functions, which include planning, abstract thinking, rule acquisition, cognitive flexibility, initiation of appropriate actions, and inhibition of inappropriate actions [291].

In general, the HD symptoms begin between 30 and 50 years of age but can start at any age [291, 292]. Approximately 8% of HD cases start before the age of 20 years, and typically present with symptoms like Parkinson's disease [291]. The worldwide HD prevalence is nearly 5 to 10 cases per 100,000 persons [293], but varies greatly geographically because of ethnicity, local migration and past immigration patterns. The HD prevalence is similar for men and women. The most common complications that reduce the life expectancy are lung (pneumonia) and cardiac diseases, and physical injury caused by falls [291]. Death due to HD typically occurs between 15 to 20 years from when this disease was first detected [291].

Although the causes of HD are not fully understood, it has been proposed that this neurodegenerative disease is primarily caused by an autosomal dominant mutation in either of an individual's two copies of a gene called Huntingtin or HTT gene [291-294]. The HTT gene provides the genetic information for HTT protein [291-294]. This protein is expressed in all mammalian cells, interacts with over 100 other proteins, and appears to have multiple biological functions [295]. However, its function in humans is yet unclear. Studies performed in animals genetically modified to exhibit HD showed that the HTT protein is important for embryonic development, and its absence is related to an embryonic death [292, 294]. It is well established that the HTT protein interacts with proteins which are involved in several cellular processes, including intracellular signalling and transporting, and gene transcription [291-294]. It was shown that the HTT protein participates in neurotransmitter vesicular transport, facilitating the synaptic neurotransmission [296].

The behavior of the mutant HTT protein is not completely understood, but it is toxic to certain cell types, particularly in the brain neurons [295]. Early brain damage likely related to the mutant HTT protein observed in HD patients is most evident in the striatum, but with the progress of HD, other areas of the brain are also more conspicuously affected [295]. Early HD symptoms are attributable to an abnormal function of the striatum and its cortical connections, namely control over movement, mood and higher cognitive function [292]. Recent studies indicated that the DNA methylation also appears to be changed in HD [297].

Several pathways, by which the mutant HTT gene may cause a neuronal death, have been identified [292, 294]. These include: (1) effects on chaperone proteins, which help fold proteins and remove misfolded ones; (2) interactions with caspases (apoptotic proteins), which play a role in the process of removing cells; (3) the toxic effects of glutamine on neuronal cells; (4) impairment of energy production within cells; and (5) effects on the expression of genes [298]. The mutant HTT gene activates the caspases through damaging the ubiquitin-protease system [292, 294]. The mutant

HTT gene also acts as an anti-apoptotic agent preventing programmed cell death and controls the production of the brain-derived neurotrophic factor (BDNF), a protein which protects neurons and regulates their creation during neurogenesis [292, 294].

If the expression of HTT protein is increased and more HTT is produced, brain survival is improved and the effects of mutant HTT gene are reduced, whereas when the expression of HTT is reduced, the resulting characteristics are more typical of the presence of the mutant HTT [296]. The disruption of the normal HTT gene appears to not cause the human HD [292]. It is thought that the human HD is also not caused by an inadequate production of the HTT protein, but by a gain of toxic function of the mutant HTT [292]. Thus, the detection of the mutant HTT gene has been used as a biomarker for diagnosis of HD in humans.

There is no cure for human HD. The treatments can relieve some symptoms, and in some, improve the quality of life. Studies on the pathogenic mechanisms of HD have focused on identifying the functioning of HTT protein, and the brain pathology that the disease produces. These studies are being conducted on many different approaches to prevent HD or slow its progression. The therapeutic strategies can be broadly grouped into three categories: (1) reduction of the mutant HTT protein levels (including gene splicing and gene silencing); (2) improvement of the neuronal survival by reducing the harm caused by the protein into specific cellular pathways and mechanisms (including protein homeostasis and histone deacetylase inhibition); (3) replacement of the death neurons using stem cells therapy.

Several pharmacological agents have been used to treat HD symptoms, including creatine, riluzole, dimebon, phenylbutyrate minocycline, ethyl-EPA, coenzyme Q10 and others. However, these drugs have been ineffective to prevent or slow the progression of human HD [291]. Satisfactory results to the treatment of the motor dysfunctions have been obtained using tetrabenazine [291]. Benzodiazepines and neuroleptics have been used to reduce chorea in HD patients. Selective serotonin reuptake inhibitors and mirtazapine have been used to treat depression in these patients, while atypical antipsychotic drugs are used to treat psychosis and behavioral problems. The antiparkinsonism drugs have been used to treat hypokinesia and rigidity. Still under investigation, preliminary positive results have been obtained using amantadine and remacemide. The HD represents a major medical, social, financial and scientific problem, but despite enormous research efforts, this disease is still incurable, and only symptomatic relief drugs are available. Thus, new approaches and targets are needed.

Although the primary dysfunctions that lead to a neurodegeneration, and neuronal death, in the brain of HD patients are not fully understood, recent evidences indicate that an abnormal calcium (Ca^{2+}) signalling in neuronal cells is involved in many of the neurodegenerative disorders, including Alzheimer's (AD) and Parkinson's (PD) diseases [261, 262]. Ca^{2+} is a ubiquitous second messenger that regulates various activities in the eukaryotic cells. Neuronal cells require extremely precise spatial-temporal control of Ca^{2+}-dependent processes because they regulate such vital functions, as synaptic plasticity. An imbalance of the intracellular Ca^{2+} homeostasis in neuronal cells could result into cytosolic Ca^{2+} overload that leads into loss of function, and neuronal death, typically observed in the neurodegenerative disorders, such as in AD and PD [261, 262]. Thus, protecting neurons from loss of function, and neuronal death, has become a promising strategy in the treatment of neurodegenerative diseases, including HD. The pharmacological modulation of the intracellular Ca^{2+} homeostasis became the major focus of the neuroprotective strategy for neurodegenerative diseases.

Ca^{2+} is a highly versatile intracellular second messenger in the neuronal cells, and regulates many complicated cellular processes, including the excitation, plasticity and apoptosis [6, 14, 15, 264-290]. Ca^{2+} influx from the extracellular fluid is required for a sustained elevation of the cytosolic Ca^{2+} concentration (($Ca^{2+})_c$), and a full activation of the Ca^{2+}-dependent processes. Voltage-activated Ca^{2+} channels (VACC) serve as the principal routes of a Ca^{2+} entry into the electrically excitable cells such as neurons. The nervous system expresses VACC with unique cellular and subcellular distribution, and specific functions. N-, P/Q- and L-type VACC are distributed at neuronal cells regulating the neuronal excitability, the neurotransmitter release, and gene expression [6, 14, 15, 264-290]. Evidences obtained from natural mutants, knockout mice, and human genetic disorders indicate a fundamental role of some VACC in a wide variety of the neurodegenerative disorders, including AD and PD [6, 14, 15, 264-290].

In addition to Ca^{2+}, other intracellular messengers are involved in the regulation of neuronal functions, including 3′-5′-cyclic adenosine monophosphate (cAMP). cAMP is a second messenger that regulates key cellular responses, including central metabolic events, cell growth, survival and differentiation, secretory processes, as well as inflammatory responses [6, 14, 15, 264-290]. Given these pleiotropic actions of cAMP, it is not surprising that the pharmaceutical manipulation of the cAMP levels in the cells has proven a therapeutic benefit in a wide range of human diseases. Investigations into the mechanisms of the cAMP signalling therefore have far reaching implications into the understanding and treatment of human diseases. It has now been over 10 years since efforts to completely understand the signalling actions of cAMP led to the discovery of the exchange protein directly activated by cAMP (EPAC) proteins [6, 14, 15, 264-290].

It has been known for some time that drugs that elevate the intracellular cAMP concentration (($cAMP)_c$), namely cAMP-enhancer compounds, have proven a therapeutic benefit for diseases ranging from depression to inflammation [6, 14, 15, 264-290]. The challenge now is to determine which of these positive actions of cAMP involve the activation of the EPAC-regulated signal transduction pathways. EPACs are specific guanine nucleotide exchange factors for the Ras GTPase homologues, Rap1 and Rap2, which they activate independently of the classical routes for cAMP signalling, cyclic nucleotide-gated ion channels and protein kinase A [6, 14, 15, 264-290]. Rather, EPAC activation is triggered by internal conformational changes induced by a direct interaction with cAMP. Leading from this has been the development of EPAC-specific agonists, which has helped to delineate numerous cellular actions of cAMP that rely on the subsequent activation of EPAC. These include regulation of the exocytosis and the control of cell adhesion, growth, division and differentiation. Recent work also implicates EPAC in the regulation of anti-inflammatory signalling in the vascular endothelium, namely negative regulation of proinflammatory cytokine signalling, and a positive support of the barrier function. Further elucidation of these important signalling mechanisms will no doubt support the development of the next generation of anti-inflammatory drugs. In addition, there is evidence that the increase of neuronal cAMP can stimulate the cellular survival pathways, and neuroregeneration, then resulting in neuroprotection [6, 14, 15, 264-290].

Evidences suggest that the dysregulation of the intracellular signalling pathways mediated by these universal regulators of cell function, Ca^{2+} and cAMP, could be implicated in the pathogenesis of the neurodegenerative diseases [6, 14, 15, 264-290]. Our previous studies have indicated that the functional interaction between the intracellular signalling pathways mediated by Ca^{2+} and cAMP [Ca^{2+}/cAMP signalling interaction] participates in several cellular responses, including in neurotransmitter and in hormone exocytosis, and in neuronal survival [6, 14, 15, 264-290]. These studies have also indicated that the pharmacological modulation of the Ca^{2+}/cAMP signalling interaction by the combined use of the Ca^{2+} channel blockers (CCB) and drugs that increment the cAMP-enhancer compounds, such as phosphodiesterase (PDE) inhibitors, can increase the neurotransmission, and additionally can stimulate a neuroprotective response in the neurodegenerative diseases [6, 14, 15, 264-290].

5.1.6. Spinal Muscular Atrophy (SMA)

It is well established that the Ca^{2+}/cAMP signalling interaction is a key cellular process in mammalians [6, 14, 15, 264-290]. This nowadays accepted concept assumes that these signalling pathways virtually exist in all mammalian cells, regulated by the adenylyl cyclases (ACs) and the phosphodiesterases (PDEs) [6, 14, 15, 264-290]. Indeed, the endoplasmic reticulum (ER) Ca^{2+} channels, notably the Ca^{2+} channels regulated by the ryanodine receptors (RyR), have particularly been a forefront for the Ca^{2+}/cAMP signalling interaction field. We recognized that the Ca^{2+}/cAMP signalling interaction plays an important participation in the regulation of transmitter release from neurons and neuroendocrine cells, and yet neuronal death originated from the neurodegenerative diseases [6, 14, 15, 264-290]. Then, the interaction of the Ca^{2+} and cAMP signalling pathways could be a new therapeutic goal for pharmaceuticals to treat the neurodegenerative diseases like spinal muscular atrophy. This disease refers to a group of disorders affecting the lower motor neurons. The age of onset of these disorders is variable, ranging from the neonatal period to adulthood. Over the last few years, there has been enormous progress in the description of new genes and phenotypes that throw new light into the molecular pathways involved in the motor neuron degeneration. Advances in our understanding of the pathophysiology of the most frequent forms, spinal muscular atrophy linked to SMN1 gene mutations and Kennedy disease, have led to the development of therapeutic strategies currently being tested in clinical trials [299]. Thus, this book discusses how the pharmacological modulation of the Ca^{2+}/cAMP signalling interaction could be a new therapeutic strategy for treating spinal muscular atrophy. Several medical reports have been proving that the prescription of the L-type CCBs in the antihypertensive therapy alleviates hypertension but produces a sympathetic hyperactivity [1]. Despite these adverse effects of the CCBs have been initially attributed to the adjust reflex of the arterial pressure, during almost four decades this enigmatic phenomenon named "calcium paradox" remained without an additional explanation. The year of 2013 would change this history forever! Through an original experiment, we revealed that the increased transmitter release from sympathetic neurons induced by the CCBs is due to their interference on the Ca^{2+}/cAMP signalling interaction, thus resulting on a "calcium paradox" phenomenon [6]. We confirmed that the contractions of the vas deferens were completely abolished by the L-type CCBs in high concentrations (>1 μmol/L), but paradoxically increased in concentrations below 1 μmol/L, thus defined as a sympathetic hyperactivity promoted by CCBs [10-12]. Our studies clearly established that the paradoxical sympathetic hyperactivity is due to an augmentation of neurotransmitter release from sympathetic neurons achieved by the L-type CCBs due to their interference on the Ca^{2+}/cAMP signalling interaction.

Indeed, many reports have shown that an elevation of cytosolic cAMP concentration ((cAMP)c) reduces the neuronal death triggered by a cytosolic

Ca^{2+} overload, then stimulating a neuroprotective effect [300, 301]. As mentioned above, the L-type CCBs increase the neurotransmitter release due to their interference on the Ca^{2+}/cAMP signalling interaction. This interference results in the increase of ACs activity and in an elevation of (cAMP)c that, in turn, stimulates a Ca^{2+} release from the ER, that increases the neurotransmitter release [6, 14, 15, 264-290]. In addition, this elevation of (cAMP)$_c$ produces neuroprotective effects mediated by the Ca^{2+}/cAMP signalling interaction. It was proposed that this neuroprotective effect results from an activation by cAMP on the cellular survival pathways mediated by PKA/CREB [6, 14, 15, 264-290]. Then, a new pharmacological goal for increasing the neurotransmission in neurological and psychiatric disorders resulting from neurotransmitter release deficit, and neuronal death, could be achieved by the pharmacological interference on the Ca^{2+}/cAMP signalling interaction. The combined use of the L-type CCBs, prescribed in the antihypertensive therapy, and (cAMP)$_c$-enhancer compounds, prescribed in the anti-depressive therapy such as rolipram, could be useful to achieve this purpose. It is important to note that the effect of this combined therapy in attenuating neuronal death may be related to a genomic response, as the synaptic release may be attributed to a rapid response. Indeed, a pharmacological modulation of the Ca^{2+}/cAMP signalling interaction by a combination of the L-type CCBs, and cAMP-enhancer drugs, could increase the neurotransmission (e.g., associated to the control of cognitive function). In addition, a pharmacological modulation of this interaction could subsidize the reducing of the neuronal death due to an attenuation of cytosolic Ca^{2+} overload, increase of (cAMP)$_c$, and stimulation of cellular survival pathways mediated by a genomic response due to the activation of cellular survival pathways regulated by the cAMP/PKA/CREB-dependent intracellular signalling pathway [261, 262, 302, 303]. Figure 5.1 illustrates how to produce cellular responses: increase of the neurotransmitter release (rapid response), and attenuation of the neuronal death (genomic response), by the pharmacological modulation of the Ca^{2+}/cAMP signalling interaction.

In fact, it was demonstrated that the prescription of the L-type CCBs reduces motor symptoms and reduces the progressive neuronal death in animal model of Parkinson's disease, indicating that the L-type CCBs are potentially viable neuroprotective pharmaceuticals [261]. Intriguingly, a 1-decade study involving thousands of senile hypertensive patients demonstrated that the prescription of L-type CCBs reduced blood pressure and the risk of dementia in hypertensive patients, indicating that these pharmaceuticals could be clinically used to treat neurodegenerative diseases [262]. These results for the neuroprotective effects of CCBs have been reinvestigated in thousands of elderly hypertensive patients with memory dysfunction [302]. These studies concluded that the patients who had taken CCBs had their risk of cognitive dysfunction decreased, such as in Alzheimer's disease [302]. These findings reinforce the idea that the reduction of cytosolic Ca^{2+} overload produced by the L-type CCBs due to a blockade of Ca^{2+} influx could be an alternative pharmacological goal to reduce, or to prevent, neuronal death in the neurodegenerative diseases like in spinal muscular atrophy. This disease is a genetic disorder that affects the control of the muscle movement. It is caused by a loss, neuronal death, of specialized nerve cells, the motor neurons. The loss of the motor neurons leads into weakness and wasting, atrophy, of muscles used for activities such as crawling, walking, sitting up, and controlling of head movement. In severe cases of spinal muscular atrophy, the muscles used for breathing and swallowing are affected. There are many types of spinal muscular atrophy distinguished by the pattern of features, severity of muscle weakness, and aging when the muscle problems begin. Based on previous described findings, we have anticipated a new therapeutic goal for increasing the neurotransmission in the neurological and psychiatric disorders resulting from neurotransmitter release deficit, and neuronal death, such as in spinal muscular atrophy [6, 14, 15, 264-290]: the pharmacological regulation of the Ca^{2+}/cAMP signalling interaction produced by the combined use of the L-type CCBs and $(cAMP)_c$-enhancer compounds, which could open a new pathway to the drug development for the treatment of spinal muscular atrophy and other neurodegenerative diseases [6, 14, 15, 264-290].

For understanding the role of the Ca^{2+}/cAMP signalling interaction in the regulation of the neuronal cells initially proposed by Bergantin and Caricati-Neto [6, 14, 15, 264-290], we should return into the past. Indeed, the concept of the stimulus-secretion to explain the neurotransmitter release has been achieved from ingenious experiments performed in the 1960s [63]. From their concepts, it was shown in the 1970s that an increase in the $(Ca^{2+})c$ is a fundamental requirement to start the transmitter release [119]. In addition, the unquestionable result showing a direct relationship between the neurotransmitter release and an elevation in $(Ca^{2+})c$ came from the fundamental experiments made by the Nobel laureate Erwin Neher [121]. Thus, by reducing the Ca^{2+} influx by blocking the voltage activated-calcium channels (VACC), we should have a reducing in the neurotransmitter release. However, many *in vitro* studies have demonstrated that selective blockers of the L-type VACC, such as nifedipine and verapamil, could induce the neurotransmitter release when used in concentrations below 1 μmol/L [10-12]. In addition, many *in vitro* studies have demonstrated that the elevation of $(cAMP)c$ enhances the transmitter release at several synapses in the autonomic nervous system of mammalians [83]. These findings decisively contributed to our discovery that the functional interaction between the intracellular signalling pathways mediated by Ca^{2+} and cAMP, named by us as Ca^{2+}/cAMP signalling interaction, participates in several cellular responses in mammalians cells, including in the neurotransmitter and hormone exocytosis, and in the neuronal survival [6, 14, 15, 264-290].

This nowadays accepted concept assumes that the Ca^{2+}/cAMP signalling interaction virtually exists in all mammalian cells, regulated by the adenylyl cyclases (AC) and the PDE [6, 14, 15, 264-290]. Indeed, the endoplasmic reticulum (ER) Ca^{2+} channels, notably the Ca^{2+} channels regulated by the ryanodine receptors (RyR), have particularly been a forefront for the Ca^{2+}/cAMP signalling interaction field. We recognized that the Ca^{2+}/cAMP signalling interaction plays an important participation in the regulation of transmitter release from neurons and neuroendocrine cells, and yet in the neuronal death originated from the neurodegenerative diseases [6, 14, 15, 264-290]. Then, the Ca^{2+}/cAMP signalling interaction could be a new therapeutic goal for pharmaceuticals to treat neurodegenerative diseases like in spinal muscular atrophy.

Several medical reports have been proving that the L-type CCBs, currently used in the antihypertensive therapy, alleviate systemic arterial hypertension due to relaxing the smooth muscle (vasodilation) of resistance arteries, but produce tachycardia and an increase of catecholamine serum levels, characterizing a CCB-induced sympathetic hyperactivity [1]. Despite these adverse effects of CCBs have been initially attributed to an adjust reflex of arterial pressure, during almost four decades this enigmatic phenomenon named "calcium paradox" remained without an additional explanation. However, this enigmatic phenomenon was also observed in *in vitro* studies, indicating that this sympathetic hyperactivity was due to a direct action of the CCB [10-12].

Using a smooth muscle richly innervated by sympathetic nerves (rat vas deferens) as a study model of the sympathetic neurotransmission, we discovered that the contractile responses mediated by sympathetic neurons were completely abolished by L-type CCB in high concentrations (>1 µmol/L) due to a selective and effective blockade of the L-type VACC but were paradoxically increased in concentrations below 1 µmol/L, confirming a CCB-induced sympathetic hyperactivity [6, 14, 15, 264-290]. Our studies initiated in 2013 clearly demonstrated that this paradoxical sympathetic hyperactivity results from the augmentation of the transmitter release from sympathetic neurons, and adrenal chromaffin cells, produced by the L-type CCB due to their interference on the Ca^{2+}/cAMP signalling interaction [6, 14, 15, 264-290]. We discovered that in low concentration, the L-type CCB produce a moderate blockade of the L-type VACC, that reduces the Ca^{2+} influx and $(Ca^{2+})_c$, that in turn attenuates an inhibitory action of Ca^{2+} on the AC, and increases the $(cAMP)_c$ synthesis, stimulating the intracellular signalling pathways mediated by cAMP [6, 14, 15, 264-290]. This Ca^{2+}/cAMP signalling interaction stimulates the Ca^{2+} release from the ER that increases the neurotransmitter release, facilitating the neurotransmission in sympathetic synapses [6, 14, 15, 264-290].

Indeed, many reports have shown that an elevation of $(cAMP)_c$ reduces the neuronal death triggered by a cytosolic Ca^{2+} overload, stimulating a neuroprotective response [300, 301]. Our studies revealed that this neuroprotective response is mediated by the Ca^{2+}/cAMP signalling interaction, that regulates the cellular survival pathways mediated by cAMP/PKA/CREB [6, 14, 15, 264-290]. Then, a new pharmacological goal for increasing neurotransmission in the neurodegenerative diseases resulting in neurotransmitter release deficit, and neuronal death, could be achieved by the pharmacological modulation of the Ca^{2+}/cAMP signalling interaction. We have proposed that the combined use of the L-type CCB, prescribed in the antihypertensive therapy such as nifedipine analogous, and cAMP-enhancer compounds, prescribed in the antidepressive therapy such as rolipram, could be useful to achieve this purpose.

It is important to note that the effect of this combined therapy in attenuating neuronal death may be related to the genomic response, as the synaptic release may be attributed to a rapid response. Indeed, a pharmacological modulation of the Ca^{2+}/cAMP signalling interaction by the combination of the L-type CCB, and cAMP-enhancer compounds, could increase the neurotransmission. In addition, the pharmacological modulation of this interaction could subsidize the reducing of neuronal death due to an attenuation of cytosolic Ca^{2+} overload, increase of $(cAMP)_c$, and stimulation of the cellular survival pathways mediated by a genomic response due to an activation of cellular survival pathways regulated by cAMP/PKA/CREB-dependent intracellular signalling pathway [261, 262, 302, 303]. Figure 5.1 illustrates how the pharmacological modulation of the Ca^{2+}/cAMP signalling interaction could produce the increase of neurotransmitter release (rapid response), and the attenuation of neuronal death (genomic response).

5.1.7. Vascular Dementia (VD)

Older people with dementia exist in nearly every country in the world. Dementia rates are predicted to increase at an alarming rate in the least developed and developing regions of the world, despite mortality resulting from the malnutrition, poverty, war, and infectious diseases. WHO projections suggest that by 2025, about three-quarters of the estimated 1.2 billion people aged 60 years and older will reside in the developing countries. Thus, by 2040, if growth in the older population continues, and considering no changes in the mortality or burden reduction by preventive measures, 71% of 81.1 million dementia cases will be in the developing world.

There are no known curative or preventive measures for the most types of dementia. Diet and lifestyle could influence the risk, and studies suggest that a midlife history of disorders that affect the vascular system, such as hypertension, type 2 diabetes, and obesity increase the risk of dementia, including AD. Increased trends in the demographic transition and urbanization within many developing countries are predicted to lead into lifestyle changes. Delaying of onset, by modifying the risk or lifestyle, decreases the prevalence and public health burden of dementia; a delay in onset of 1 year would translate into almost a million fewer prevalent cases in the USA. However, this in turn might increase demands on health services and costs for the older populations.

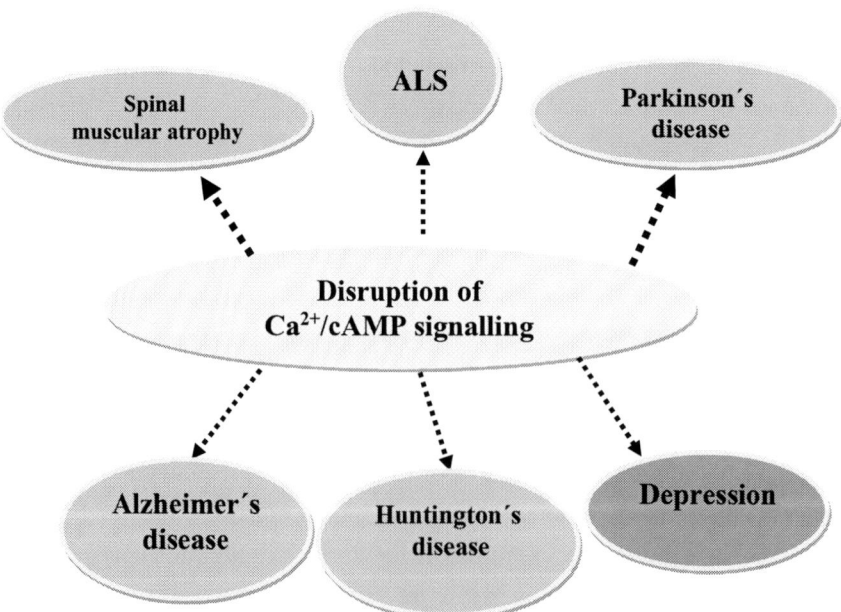

Figure 5.1. Disruption of Ca^{2+}/cAMP signalling and its consequences.
ALS: amyotrophic lateral sclerosis.

VD and AD are progressive neurodegenerative disorders related to aging characterized by a cognitive and memory deterioration. VD is one of the most common causes of dementia after AD, causing around 15% of the cases. However, unlike AD, there are no licensed treatments for VD. Progress in the specialty has been difficult because of uncertainties over the disease classification and diagnostic criteria, controversy over the exact nature of the relation between cerebrovascular pathology and a cognitive impairment, and the paucity of identifiable tractable treatment targets. Although there is an established relation between vascular and the degenerative AD pathology, the mechanistic link between the two has not yet been identified.

VD is recognized as the second most prevalent type of dementia. Subcortical VD caused by a small-artery disease, associated with hypertensive disease, seems to be a common (73%) cause of VD. In AD, neuritic plaques represent the pathological status of this dementia type and are respectively related to the accumulation of the β-amyloid peptide (Aβ) in the brain tissues [248, 304]. The neurotoxic potential of the Aβ results from its biochemical properties that favor an aggregation. These processes, along with a reduction of Aβ clearance from the brain, lead to the extracellular accumulation of Aβ, and the subsequent activation of neurotoxic cascades that ultimately lead to cytoskeletal changes, neuronal dysfunction and cellular death [304]. Therapies targeting the modification of amyloid-related cascades may be viewed as promising strategies to attenuate or even to prevent dementia [304]. The inhibition of ACh degradation by AChE has been an important target to treat AD [249, 251, 305]. Therefore, the cumulative knowledge on the pathogenesis of different types of dementia derived from basic science models will hopefully be translated into a clinical practice in the forthcoming years.

It is well established that an imbalance of the intracellular Ca^{2+} homeostasis decisively contributes to the pathogenesis of aging-related neurodegenerative diseases, including VD and AD. Several evidences suggest that aging impairs the ability of the brain intracellular Ca^{2+} homeostasis, which is likely to induce a cellular damage due to a cytosolic Ca^{2+} overload, leading to a neural death and resulting into cognitive dysfunction, such as in VD and AD. Therefore, the regulation of the intracellular Ca^{2+} homeostasis may represent a new strategy for the treatment of VD and AD.

A 10-year follow-up study (2000 to 2010), involving 82,107 hypertensive patients of more than 60 years of age, showed that the use of L-type CCBs reduced the blood pressure and the risk of dementia in hypertensives, suggesting that these drugs could be clinically used to treat VD and AD [262]. Supportive findings for the neuroprotective effects of CCBs have been demonstrated in 1,241 elderly hypertensive patients with memory impairment [302]. The use of CCBs decreased the risk of cognitive impairment and AD independently of the BP levels, when compared to patients not receiving the CCBs [302]. The long-term effects of the antihypertensive therapy, initiated with a long-acting dihydropyridine (nitrendipine), have been demonstrated in the double-blind, placebo-controlled Syst-Eur trial, in which the incidence of dementia was reduced by 55%.

Some studies have proposed that hybrid compounds having the moieties of tacrine, a potent inhibitor of brain and peripheral AChE, and nimodipine, a L-type CCB could be useful to the treatment of AD [249, 251]. In addition, galantamine, a mild AChE inhibitor and an allosteric ligand of nicotinic receptors has been used to improve cognition and behavior in patients with AD [305].

It was shown in dementia model rats that the cAMP-enhancer compounds, such as nobiletin (a polymethoxylated flavone from citrus peels) and oxyntomodulin (a proglucagon-derived peptide that co-activates the GLP-1 receptor and the glucagon receptor) produce a neuroprotective effect mediated by the intracellular cAMP production, activation of PKA and MAPK pathways, and phosphorylation of CREB [303, 306].

Our discovery of the involvement of the Ca^{2+}/cAMP signalling interaction in the neurotransmission and neuroprotection has produced important advances in the understanding of the pathophysiology and pharmacology of VD and AD [6, 14, 15, 264-290]. These advances allowed us to propose that the pharmacological modulation of the Ca^{2+}/cAMP signalling interaction produced by a combined use of the L-type CCBs (used in the antihypertensive therapy), such as isradipine, and cAMP-enhancer compounds (used in the anti-depressive therapy), such as rolipram could represent a new therapeutic strategy for the treatment of VD and AD in humans.

Pharmacological modulation of the Ca^{2+}/cAMP signalling interaction by a combined use of the L-type CCBs and cAMP-enhancer drugs could attenuate the ACh release deficit, increasing the central cholinergic neurotransmission involved in the control of cognitive function [6, 14, 15, 264-290]. In addition, the pharmacological modulation of this interaction could contribute to reduce the neuronal death due to attenuation of the cytosolic Ca^{2+} overload, increase of $(cAMP)_c$ and stimulation of the cellular survival pathways probably mediated by an activation of the cellular survival pathways regulated by AMP/PKA/CREB-dependent intracellular signalling pathways [300, 301, 303, 306]. Thus, a pharmacological modulation of the Ca^{2+}/cAMP signalling interaction could be a new neuroprotective therapeutic strategy to slow the progression of VD and AD [6, 14, 15, 264-290].

Chapter 6

THE PHARMACOLOGICAL MODULATION OF THE CA^{2+}/CAMP SIGNALLING INTERACTION AS A THERAPEUTIC STRATEGY FOR NEUROLOGICAL AND PSYCHIATRIC DISEASES: A THEORY AND SUPPORTING DATA

For understanding the role of the Ca^{2+}/cAMP signalling interaction in the regulation of the neuronal cells initially proposed by Bergantin et al. [6, 14, 15, 264-290], we should return into the past. Indeed, the concept of a stimulus-secretion to explain the neurotransmitter release has been achieved from ingenious experiments performed in the 1960s [63]. From their concepts, it was shown in the 1970s that an increase in the (Ca^{2+})c is a fundamental requirement to start a transmitter release [119]. In addition, the unquestionable result showing a direct relationship between the neurotransmitter release and an elevation in (Ca^{2+})c came from the fundamental experiments made by the Nobel laureate Erwin Neher. Thus, by reducing the Ca^{2+} influx by blocking the VACC, we should have a reducing in the neurotransmitter release. However, many *in vitro* studies have demonstrated that the selective blockers of the L-type VACC, such as nifedipine and verapamil, could induce the neurotransmitter release when used in concentrations below 1 µmol/L [10-12]. In addition, many *in vitro* studies have demonstrated that the elevation of $(cAMP)_c$ enhances the transmitter release at several synapses in the autonomic nervous system of mammalians [83]. These findings decisively contributed to our discovery that the functional interaction between the intracellular signalling pathways mediated by Ca^{2+} and cAMP, namely by us as $Ca^{2+}/cAMP$ signalling interaction, participates in several cellular responses in mammalians cells, including the neurotransmitter and hormone exocytosis, and yet neuronal survival [6, 14, 15, 264-290].

This nowadays accepted concept assumes that the $Ca^{2+}/cAMP$ signalling interaction virtually exists in all mammalian cells, regulated by the adenylyl cyclases (AC) and the PDE [6, 14, 15, 264-290]. Indeed, the endoplasmic reticulum (ER) Ca^{2+} channels, notably the Ca^{2+} channels regulated by the ryanodine receptors (RyR), have particularly been a forefront for the $Ca^{2+}/cAMP$ signalling interaction field. We recognized that the $Ca^{2+}/cAMP$ signalling interaction plays an important role in the regulation of the transmitter release from neurons and neuroendocrine cells, and yet neuronal death originated from the neurodegenerative diseases [6, 14, 15, 264-290]. Then, the $Ca^{2+}/cAMP$ signalling interaction could be a new therapeutic goal for pharmaceuticals to treat the neurodegenerative diseases like HD, and others.

Several medical reports have been proving that the L-type CCBs, currently used in the antihypertensive therapy, alleviate systemic arterial hypertension due to relaxing the smooth muscle (vasodilation) of resistance arteries, but produce tachycardia and an increase of catecholamine serum levels, then characterizing a CCB-induced sympathetic hyperactivity [1]. Despite these adverse effects of CCB having been initially attributed to adjusting the reflex of arterial pressure, during almost four decades this enigmatic phenomenon named "calcium paradox" remained without an additional explanation. However, this enigmatic phenomenon was also observed from *in vitro* studies, indicating that this sympathetic hyperactivity was due to a direct action of the CCB [10-12].

Using a smooth muscle richly innervated by sympathetic nerves (rat vas deferens) as a study model of the sympathetic neurotransmission, we discovered that the contractile responses mediated by the sympathetic neurons were completely abolished by the L-type CCB in high concentrations (>1 µmol/L) due to a selective, and effective, blockade of the L-type VACC but were paradoxically increased in concentrations below 1 µmol/L, confirming a CCB-induced sympathetic hyperactivity [6, 14, 15, 264-290]. Our studies initiated in 2013 clearly demonstrated that this paradoxical sympathetic hyperactivity results from the augmentation of the transmitter release from sympathetic neurons, and adrenal chromaffin cells, produced by the L-type CCB due to their interference on the Ca^{2+}/cAMP signalling interaction [6, 14, 15, 264-290]. We discovered that in low concentration, the L-type CCB produce a moderate blockade of the L-type VACC, that reduces the Ca^{2+} influx and $(Ca^{2+})c$, that in turn attenuates an inhibitory action of Ca^{2+} on the AC, and increases the $(cAMP)_c$ synthesis, stimulating the intracellular signalling pathways mediated by cAMP [6, 14, 15, 264-290]. This Ca^{2+}/cAMP signalling interaction stimulates a Ca^{2+} release from the ER that increases the neurotransmitter release, facilitating the neurotransmission in sympathetic synapses [6, 14, 15, 264-290].

Indeed, many reports have shown that an elevation of $(cAMP)c$ reduces the neuronal death triggered by a cytosolic Ca^{2+} overload, stimulating a neuroprotective response [300, 301]. Our studies revealed that this neuroprotective response is mediated by the Ca^{2+}/cAMP signalling interaction that regulates the cellular survival pathways mediated by cAMP/PKA/CREB [6, 14, 15, 264-290]. Then, a new pharmacological goal for increasing the neurotransmission in the neurodegenerative diseases resulting from neurotransmitter release deficit, and neuronal death, could be achieved by the pharmacological modulation of the Ca^{2+}/cAMP signalling interaction. We have proposed that the combined use of the L-type CCB, prescribed in the antihypertensive therapy such as nifedipine analogous, and cAMP-enhancer compounds, prescribed in the antidepressive therapy such as rolipram, could be useful to achieve this purpose.

It is important to note that the effect of this combined therapy in attenuating neuronal death may be related to the genomic response, as the synaptic release may be attributed to a rapid response. Indeed, a pharmacological modulation of the Ca^{2+}/cAMP signalling interaction by the combination of the L-type CCB, and cAMP-enhancer compounds, could increase the neurotransmission. In addition, a pharmacological modulation of this interaction could subsidize the reducing of neuronal death due to an attenuation of the cytosolic Ca^{2+} overload, increase of $(cAMP)_c$, and stimulation of the cell survival pathways mediated by a genomic response due to an activation of cellular survival pathways regulated by cAMP/PKA/CREB-dependent intracellular signalling pathways [261, 262, 302, 303]. Figure 8.1 illustrates how the pharmacological modulation of the Ca^{2+}/cAMP signalling interaction could produce the increase of neurotransmitter release (rapid response), and the attenuation of the neuronal death (genomic response).

The known genetic cause of HD has fueled considerable progress in the understanding of its pathobiology, and the development of therapeutic approaches aimed at correcting specific changes linked to the causative mutation. Among the most promising is reducing the expression of the mutant HTT protein with RNA interference or antisense oligonucleotides; human trials are now being planned. Zinc-finger transcriptional repression is another innovative method to reduce the mutant HTT protein expression. Modulation of the mutant HTT protein phosphorylation, chaperone upregulation, and autophagy enhancement represent attempts to alter the cellular homeostasis to favor removal of the mutant HTT protein. Inhibition of histone deacetylases (HDACs) remains of interest; with several approaches being pursued, including a BDNF mimesis through the tyrosine receptor kinase B (TrkB) agonism and monoclonal antibodies. An increasing understanding of the role of glial cells in HD has led to several new therapeutic avenues, including a kynurenine monooxygenase inhibition, immunomodulation by the laquinimod, a CB2 agonism, and others. The complex metabolic derangements in HD remain under study, but no clear therapeutic strategy has yet emerged.

The development of new effective therapeutic strategies for HD depends on the advancement of the scientific knowledge about the primary mechanisms involved in HD pathogenesis. This can take many years and cost many millions of dollars. Thus, alternative proposal for the treatment of HD symptoms could be attempted. In fact, some studies demonstrated that the use of L-type CCB reduces neurological/psychiatric and motor symptoms in the neurodegenerative diseases, such as AD and PD [261, 262]. It was shown that the L-type CCB reduced a progressive neuronal death in animal model of PD, indicating that these drugs are potentially viable neuroprotective pharmaceuticals [261]. A 1-decade study, involving thousands of senile hypertensive patients, showed that the prescription of L-type CCB reduced both blood pressure and the risk of dementia in hypertensive patients, indicating that these pharmaceuticals could be clinically used to treat neurodegenerative diseases [262]. These results for the neuroprotective effects of CCB have been reinvestigated in thousands of elderly hypertensive patients with memory dysfunction [302]. In addition, these studies concluded that the patients who had taken CCB had their risk of cognitive dysfunction decreased, such as AD [302]. These findings reinforce the idea that the attenuation of cytosolic Ca^{2+} overload due to a blockade of Ca^{2+} influx though the L-type VACC blockade, by L-type CCB, is a pharmacological strategy to reduce, or prevent, neuronal death in the neurodegenerative diseases like HD [6, 14, 15, 264-290].

Like PD, the HD is a neurological disease resulting from neurodegenerative disorders that affects the motor control of the skeletal muscles, producing the progressive loss of motor function [291]. It is caused by a loss, neuronal death, of specialized nerve cells, the motor neurons. The loss of motor neurons leads into weakness and wasting, atrophy, of the muscles used for activities such as crawling, walking, sitting up, and controlling of the head movement [291]. In severe cases of HD, the muscles involved in breathing and swallowing are dramatically affected. Deranged cellular signalling provides several tractable targets, but the specificity and complexity are challenges. Restoring the neurotrophic support in HD remains a key potential therapeutic approach.

Altered synaptic plasticity is one potential reversible cause of dysfunction in HD. The use of the PDE inhibitors to restore the neuronal function due to an increment of the $(cAMP)_c$ has progressed rapidly into human trials [307]. Impairment of the cAMP intracellular signalling and the dysregulation of gene transcription mediated by the CREB are established features of HD [308, 309]. PDE10A is almost exclusively expressed in the striatum, and its activity is intimately linked to the synaptic biology of medium spiny neurons, whose death is a prominent feature of HD. PDE10A regulates cAMP and cyclic guanosine monophosphate (cGMP) signalling, synaptic plasticity and the response to cortical stimulation. PDE10A inhibition, or genetic deletion, induces numerous CREB–related gene expression changes and alterations in synaptic function, suggested of being beneficial in HD, and schizophrenia. Studies using R6/2 mouse showed that the PDE10A inhibition with TP-10 ameliorated motor deficits, reduced striatal atrophy and increased brain-derived neurotrophic factor (BDNF) levels. Detailed study of PDE10A, and its pharmacological inhibition, is underway to validate it as a target in HD.

One concern is that early death of striatal neurons might deplete PDE10A levels into the extent that the target is lost. However, clinical studies using PET imaging with the PDE10A radioligands, such as (18F)-MNI-695, suggest that the PDE10A levels are sufficient even in manifest HD to expect a meaningful response. Clinical studies using selective PDE10A inhibitors in HD patients are already underway, with motor and functional MRI endpoints. Studies using a R6/2 mouse showed that the selective PDE4 inhibition with rolipram, meanwhile, improved the survival and ameliorated the neuropathology and motor phenotypes.

Many exciting therapeutics are progressing through the development of new neuroprotective pharmacological strategies; then, combining a better understanding of HD biology in human patients with concerted medicinal chemistry efforts will be crucial for bringing about an era of effective therapies. Based in previous studies [6, 14, 15, 264-290], we have proposed that the pharmacological modulation of the Ca^{2+}/cAMP signalling interaction by the combined use of the CCB and cAMP-enhancer compounds could open a new avenue for the drug development more effective, and safer, for treating neurodegenerative diseases, including HD.

Our previous studies have indicated that the pharmacological modulation of the Ca^{2+}/cAMP signalling interaction by the combined use of the Ca^{2+} channel blockers (CCB) and drugs that increment the intracellular concentration of cAMP (cAMP-enhancer compounds) can increase the neurotransmission and stimulate a neuroprotective response in the neurodegenerative diseases. Thus, we have proposed that the pharmacological modulation of this intracellular signalling mediated by Ca^{2+} and cAMP could open a new avenue for the drug development more effective, and safer, for the treatment of the neurodegenerative diseases, including HD.

In fact, it was demonstrated that the use of L-type CCBs reduces motor symptoms and reduces a progressive neuronal death in animal model of Parkinson's disease, indicating that the L-type CCBs are potentially viable neuroprotective pharmaceuticals [261]. Intriguingly, a 1-decade study, involving thousands of senile hypertensive patients, demonstrated that the prescription of L-type CCBs reduced both blood pressure and the risk of dementia in hypertensive patients, indicating that these pharmaceuticals could be clinically used to treat neurodegenerative diseases [262]. These results for the neuroprotective effects of CCBs have been reinvestigated in thousands elderly hypertensive patients with memory dysfunction [302]. In addition, these studies concluded that the patients who have taken CCBs had their risk of cognitive dysfunction decreased, such as Alzheimer's disease [302]. Together, these findings reinforce the idea that the reduction of cytosolic Ca^{2+} overload produced by L-type CCBs due to a blockade of Ca^{2+} influx could be an alternative pharmacological goal to reduce, or prevent, a neuronal death in the neurodegenerative diseases like ALS. This neurological disease results from a neurodegenerative disorder that affects the motor control of skeletal muscles, producing the progressive loss of motor function. It is caused by a loss, neuronal death, of specialized nerve cells, the motor neurons. The loss of the motor neurons leads into weakness and wasting, atrophy, of the muscles used for activities such as crawling, walking, sitting up, and controlling of the head movement. In severe cases of ALS, the muscles involved in breathing and swallowing are dramatically affected.

Based on previous described findings, we have anticipated a new therapeutic goal for increasing the neurotransmission in neurological and psychiatric disorders like depression, resulting from the neurotransmitter release deficit and neuronal death [6, 14, 15, 264-290]: the pharmacological regulation of the Ca^{2+}/cAMP signalling interaction produced by the combined use of the L-type CCBs and cAMP-enhancer compounds (see Table 6.1), which could open a new pathway to the drug development for the treatment of ALS and other neurodegenerative diseases, and also depression [6, 14, 15, 264-290].

Table 6.1. A list of several CCBs and cAMP signalling-enhancer compounds

Ca^{2+} channel blockers (CCBs)	cAMP signalling (enhancer compounds)
Verapamil	1. Rolipram
Nifedipine	2. 3-isobutyl-1-methylxanthine (IBMX)
Diltiazem	3. Forskolin
Isradipine	4. Aminophylline
Amlodipine	5. Theophylline
Nicardipine	6. Paraxanthine

Chapter 7

PARADOXICAL EFFECTS OF THE CCB AND THEIR PLEIOTROPIC EFFECTS

Since four decades ago, several clinical studies have been reporting that an acute and chronic administration of the L-type CCB, such as nifedipine and verapamil, produces reduction in both peripheral vascular resistance and arterial pressure, associated with an increase in plasma noradrenaline levels and heart rate, typical effects of sympathetic hyperactivity [1]. However, the cellular and molecular mechanisms involved in this apparent sympathomimetic effect of the L-type CCB remained unclear for decades. In addition, experimental studies using isolated tissues richly innervated by sympathetic nerves showed that the neurogenic responses were completely inhibited by the L-type CCB in high concentrations (>1 µM), but paradoxically potentiated in concentrations below 1 µM [11, 12]. During almost four decades, these enigmatic phenomena remained unclear. In 2013, we discovered that this paradoxical increase in sympathetic activity produced by the L-type CCB is due to the Ca^{2+}/cAMP interaction [6]. Then, the pharmacological manipulation of the Ca^{2+}/cAMP interaction produced by the combination of the L-type CCB used in the antihypertensive therapy, and cAMP accumulating compounds used in the anti-depressive therapy such as rolipram, could represent a potential cardiovascular risk for hypertensive patients due to an increase in sympathetic hyperactivity.

In contrast, in 2015 we proposed that this pharmacological manipulation could be a new therapeutic strategy for increasing the neurotransmission in the psychiatric disorders, and producing neuroprotection in the neurodegenerative diseases [14]. In addition, several studies have been demonstrating pleiotropic effects of the CCB, see review [245]. CCB, like nifedipine, genuinely have pleiotropic effects [245]. Ca^{2+} channels are important regulators of the central nervous system, and their dysfunction can give rise into pathophysiological conditions as the psychiatric conditions such as epilepsy, pain and autism. In the nervous system, the CCB have been emerging as potential therapeutic avenues for pathologies such as Parkinson's and Alzheimer's disease. In fact, apart from their classical functions, CCB are described to have beneficial roles on the cognitive profile of the aged population and individuals with hypertension, diabetes, Parkinson's disease, and Alzheimer's [245]. However, the molecular mechanisms involved in these pleiotropic effects remain under debate. Different mechanisms have been proposed, but the exact mechanisms are still uncertain.

7.1. Involvement of the Ca^{2+}/cAMP Interaction: Role in the CCB Pleiotropic Effects

In Contrast To The Adverse Effects Produced By The combination of the L-type CCB with cAMP accumulating compounds in the cardiovascular diseases, the pharmacological implications of the Ca^{2+}/cAMP interaction produced by this drug combination could be used to stimulate the neuroprotection and to enhance neurotransmission [14].

Considering our model in which the increment of $(cAMP)_c$ stimulates the Ca^{2+} release from the ER (Figure 1.2), it may be reasonable the therapeutic use of the PDE inhibitor rolipram, in combination with low doses of CCB to increase the neurotransmission in the areas of central nervous system involved in neurological/psychiatric disorders, in which the neurotransmission is reduced. This new pharmacological strategy for the treatment of psychiatric disorders could increase the therapeutic efficacy and reduce the adverse effects of the medicines currently used for treating the neurological and psychiatric disorders. Considering that the CCB genuinely exhibit cognitive-enhancing abilities and reduce the risk of neurodegenerative diseases like Parkinson's and Alzheimer's diseases, and that the mechanisms involved in these pleiotropic effects are largely unknown [245]; then, whether the Ca^{2+}/cAMP interaction is involved in such effects deserves special attention. Thus, considering a $(Ca^{2+})c$ elevation could contribute to both: negatively to the neuroprotective effects and positively to the exocytosis, the therapeutic use of the PDE inhibitors may be plausible in combination with the CCB for neuroprotective purposes, and to enhance exocytosis for antidepressant purposes [14]. Then, a pharmacological interference on the Ca^{2+}/cAMP interaction produced by the combination of L-type CCB and cAMP-accumulating compounds could stimulate a neuroprotective response and reduce the clinical symptoms of the neurodegenerative diseases. Thus, the association of current medicines could enhance neurological and psychiatric disorder treatments. For example: the association of current psychiatric/neurological medicines with CCB, or rolipram, could dramatically improve the typical antidepressant, antiparkinsonism and anti-Alzheimer therapies, mainly by reducing the adverse effects and increasing the therapeutic effectiveness. Thus, this new pharmacological strategy could be alternatively used for the treatment of the symptoms of neurological and psychiatric disorders like the neurodegenerative diseases.

In conclusion, the pharmacological modulation of the Ca^{2+}/cAMP signalling interaction could be a more effective therapeutic approach for attenuating a motor neuronal death and stimulating the neuromuscular cholinergic neurotransmission compromised by an acetylcholine release deficit in ALS, and in other neurodegenerative diseases.

Chapter 8

ADDITIONAL INTERESTING FINDINGS, AND CONCEPTS, FOR THE Ca^{2+}/cAMP SIGNALLING PATHWAYS AND NEUROLOGICAL/PSYCHIATRIC DISORDERS FIELD

8.1. Ca^{2+} SIGNALLING IN HEALTHY BRAINS, AND THE EFFECTS OF AGING

As described above, the neuron uses Ca^{2+} signals to control the release of neurotransmitter, to mediate activity-dependent changes in the gene expression and to modulate a neuronal growth, the differentiation, and a transition into apoptosis [69, 70]. Neuronal Ca^{2+} signalling involves an intricate interplay between a Ca^{2+} influx across the plasma membrane through the VACC, the TRP (transient receptor potential) channels, and a Ca^{2+} release from the intracellular Ca^{2+} stores via the IP_3R, and RyR channels in the ER [121]. Intracellular Ca^{2+} release via the IP_3R is triggered by the second messenger IP_3, which is produced following an activation of metabotropic receptors coupled to the phospholipase C. Neuronal RyR functions as Ca^{2+}-activated Ca^{2+} channels which further amplifies the Ca^{2+} signals, originating from other sources [264-290]. Mitochondria also plays a significant role in shaping the neuronal Ca^{2+} signalling by utilizing potent mitochondrial Ca^{2+} uptake mechanisms [71]. Ca^{2+} uptake into mitochondria plays an important role in neuronal physiology by stimulating the mitochondrial metabolism and an increasing of mitochondrial energy production [71]. Excessive Ca^{2+} uptake into mitochondria can lead into the opening of a permeability transition pore (PTP), and into apoptosis. Owing to its importance for the neuronal function, Ca^{2+} signalling in neurons is tightly compartmentalized, and regulated within signalling microdomains which involve, for example, a functional coupling between the VACC and intracellular Ca^{2+} release channels, or between the ER Ca^{2+} release and a Ca^{2+} uptake into mitochondria [14, 28, 38]. The major risk factor for AD is an advancing age; in the most common sporadic form of AD, the individuals first manifest symptoms when they are in their 7th or 8th decades of life. But, even those who inherit a disease-causing mutation in the APP, or one of the presenilins (PS1 and PS2), remain asymptomatic into their fourth or fifth decades [310]. Age-related alterations in specific Ca^{2+}-regulating systems in brain cells have been reported, including: an elevated intracellular Ca^{2+} levels; an enhanced Ca^{2+} influx through the voltage-dependent Ca^{2+} channels; an impaired ability of mitochondria to buffer or cycle Ca^{2+}; a perturbed Ca^{2+} regulation in ryanodine and IP_3-sensitive Ca^{2+} stores. Gene array and proteomic analyses suggest a dysregulation of the expression of an array of Ca^{2+}-handling systems during aging [310]. Many of the alterations in Ca^{2+}-handling described in normal aging can be reproduced by subjecting neurons to an oxidative and metabolic stress in culture or in vivo, suggesting important contributions of these fundamental aging processes to the dysregulation of neuronal Ca^{2+} regulation in AD. Moreover, studies of brain tissue samples obtained from brains of AD patients, and animal models of AD, have revealed significant alterations in levels of proteins and genes directly involved in neuronal Ca^{2+} signalling [310].

8.2. Amyloid β-Peptide Endorses Ca^{2+} Influx and a Ca^{2+}-Mediated Excitotoxicity

As described above, amyloid plaques, a histological hallmark of AD, are comprised of extracellular aggregates of the Aβ, a 40–42 amino acid peptide generated by successive enzymatic cleavages of APP by β- and γ-secretases. Aβ is believed to be a pivotal mediator of neuronal degeneration, and an impaired cognitive function in AD [310]. Adverse effects of Aβ on synaptic function and on neuronal survival are mediated primarily by soluble protein oligomers. Aβ interaction with the plasma membrane results in an elevated $(Ca^{2+})_c$, and an increased vulnerability of the neurons to an excitotoxicity. Oligomeric forms of Aβ42 cause a Ca^{2+}-mediated toxicity in cultured cells [310]. Degenerative changes occur in neurites associated with Aβ deposits in APP mutant mice, suggesting the involvement of a Ca^{2+}-mediated Aβ neurotoxicity in vivo. In addition to an increasing of the production of Aβ, the amyloidogenic processing of APP may perturb the neuronal Ca^{2+} homeostasis by decreasing the production of a secreted form of APP (sAPPα) that activates K$^+$ channels, and by generating an APP intracellular domain that affects the ER Ca^{2+} release by regulating the expression of genes involved in Ca^{2+} homeostasis [310].

One mechanism by which Aβ may cause a Ca^{2+} influx is by inserting into the plasma membrane and forming ion-conducting pores. Neurotoxic forms of Aβ are oligomers that share a structural and a functional homology with pore-forming bacterial toxins, and the cytotoxic lymphocyte protein perforin. Interestingly, the ability of Aβ to associate with membranes and form channels is enhanced by the exposure of phosphatidylserine on the cell surface [310]. Because the cell surface exposure of phosphatidylserine is usually indicative of an apoptotic or energy-deprived cells, it is possible that the age-related mitochondrial impairments may increase the surface phosphatidylserine levels in affected neurons, and thereby facilitate a Aβ-mediated pore formation, Ca^{2+} influx and cell death; indeed, neurons with reduced cytosolic ATP levels and an elevated surface phosphatidylserine are particularly vulnerable to a Aβ toxicity. The surface exposure of the phosphatidylserine may also result from an activation of a Ca^{2+}-sensitive phospholipid scramblase 1 (PLSCR1), which mediates a rapid trans-bilayer reorganization of plasma membrane phospholipids [310].

A different mechanism by which Aβ perturbs the neuronal Ca^{2+} homeostasis is by inducing a membrane lipid peroxidation. During a peptide oligomer formation, Aβ generates a hydrogen peroxide, a process enhanced by the iron (Fe^{2+}) and copper (Cu^+). Hydrogen peroxide is then converted into a hydroxyl radical which initiates lipid peroxidation, resulting into the generation of toxic lipid aldehydes such a 4-hydroxynonenal, which impairs the function of the ion-motive ATPases, and glutamate and glucose transporters, resulting into a Ca^{2+} overload, a synaptic dysfunction, a neuronal degeneration and a cognitive impairment [310]. Particularly striking is the ability of Aβ to increase the vulnerability of neurons into excitotoxicity mediated by the N-methyl-D-aspartate (NMDA) receptor. Because excessive and sustained Ca^{2+} elevations induce a free radical production (by altering the mitochondrial oxidative phosphorylation and activating oxygenases), it is likely that the perturbed Ca^{2+} homeostasis contributes to the increased oxidative stress in neurons in AD, resulting in a self-amplifying cascade of free radical- and Ca^{2+}-mediated degenerative processes. Lesser amounts of Aβ may also be toxic to neurons. For example, exposure of rat organotypic hippocampal slice cultures to picomolar concentrations of Aβ oligomers caused the loss of dendritic spines, and decreased numbers of electrophysiologically active synapses; the spine loss was reversible and required NMDA receptor activity [310]. Aβ oligomers cause an increase in the NMDA receptor activity, which may require a direct association between the Aβ oligomers and NR1 subunit of the NMDAR. On the other hand, Aβ oligomers may suppress the activity of presynaptic P/Q-type VACC. Aβ also blocks the response of α7-containing nicotinic acetylcholine receptors (nAChRs) in hippocampal neurons, and directly evokes sustained nAChR-mediated increases in presynaptic Ca^{2+} levels, suggesting a mechanism for the impairment of cholinergic signalling in AD [264-290].

8.2.1. Presenilins

Presenilins (PS1 and the structurally and functionally related PS2) are integral membrane proteins. The holoprotein form of presenilins is located in the ER. Both PS1 and PS2 holoproteins undergo into endoproteolysis in the cytosolic loop between the 6th and 7th transmembrane domains, resulting into the generation of amino-terminal and carboxy-terminal fragments, which remain associated with each other [310]. Cleaved presenilins assemble with nicastrin, Aph-1 and Pen-2, exit from the ER and translocate into the Golgi apparatus, and eventually into plasma membrane. A mature complex of cleaved presenilins, nicastrin, Aph-1 and Pen-2 possesses aspartyl protease activity, and functions as the γ-secretase enzyme that cleaves the APP to generate the Aβ [310]. Many mutations in presenilins that cause familial (dominantly inherited) AD (FAD) increase the production of the long aggregation-prone form of Aβ (Aβ42), or reduce the production of a short soluble form, Aβ40, and therefore one way in which presenilin mutations may perturb the neuronal Ca^{2+} homeostasis is by elevating the Aβ42:Aβ40 ratio and activating the Aβ oligomer-mediated mechanisms.

Additional roles for presenilins in modulating the Ca^{2+} homeostasis is suggested by data linking two other presenilin substrate cleavage products, the AICD and the Notch intracellular domain (NICD), into a Ca^{2+}-mediated neuroplasticity and cell death. AICD may translocate into the nucleus, and therein may regulate the expression of genes encoding proteins involved in the Ca^{2+} homeostasis. Notch, a membrane receptor activated by cell surface-associated ligands such as Jagged and Delta, plays fundamental roles in regulating the proliferation and differentiation of neural progenitor cells in the developing and adult brains. Upon ligand binding, the γ-secretase cleaves Notch to release the NICD which translocates into the nucleus, where it regulates the gene transcription. Recent findings suggest potential roles for Notch and NICD in the synaptic plasticity, learning and memory, and in Ca^{2+}-mediated cell death [310].

A γ-secretase-independent connection between the presenilins and the Ca^{2+} signalling was initially suggested in Ca^{2+} imaging experiments with fibroblasts from FAD patients containing a PS1-A246E mutation [310]. It was then shown that cultured neural cells expressing AD PS1 mutations exhibit increased amounts of Ca^{2+} released from the ER, when exposed to ligands that stimulate the IP_3 production or an activation of RyR. Similar results were obtained in Ca^{2+} imaging experiments with *Xenopus* oocytes injected with cRNA encoding both PS1-M146V and PS2-N141I FAD mutants [310], in experiments with synaptosomes and cortical neurons from a PS1-M146V mutant mice [311, 312], and in hippocampal neurons from a PS2-N141I transgenic mice. In vivo studies demonstrated that the exaggerated ER Ca^{2+} signalling resulting from FAD mutations in presenilins leads into a sensitization of PS-FAD neurons to Aβ, and excitotoxic cell death via a Ca^{2+}-dependent mechanism involving an excessive Ca^{2+} release from the ER [311, 312].

Biochemical and functional interactions have been uncovered between the presenilins and several ER Ca^{2+}-regulating proteins, including the ryanodine receptors, sorcin, the myristoylated calcium-binding protein calmyrin and the calsenilin. Presenilins may also modulate the SERCA Ca^{2+} pump activity. Presenilin-2 has been reported to associate with the IP_3R to enhance the IP_3R activity. Specific effects of FAD mutants, PS1-M146V and PS2-N141I, on sensitivity of IP_3R1 to an activation by IP_3 have been recently discovered in patch-clamp experiments. A significant increase in the ryanodine receptor expression levels has been reported in brains from a PS1 mutant mice, an alteration that increases as the mice ages, providing a potential link between the AD pathogenesis and aging.

While the studies described above suggest that the FAD mutations in presenilins act by altering a normal function of other Ca^{2+}-regulating proteins, recent findings indicated that the presenilins themselves may play a direct role in Ca^{2+} signalling. It is well established that the ER membrane is "leaky" for Ca^{2+}, but the exact identity of the putative "Ca^{2+} leak channel" was previously unknown. Recent results suggest that the presenilins function as ER Ca^{2+} leak channels in the cells, and that a balance between the SERCA Ca^{2+} pump activity and the presenilin-mediated passive Ca^{2+} leak determines the steady-state resting of ER Ca^{2+} levels in the cells [310]. The ER Ca^{2+} leak function of presenilins does not involve a γ-secretase activity and is not supported by a cleaved form of presenilins; instead many FAD mutations in presenilins result into a "loss of function" for the ER Ca^{2+} leak activity, then resulting into an excessive Ca^{2+} accumulation in the ER [310]. Although most tested FAD mutants in presenilins compromised their ER Ca^{2+} leak function, the PS1-ΔE9 mutant was unique, and appeared to act as a "gain of function" leading into "super leaky" channels. The "gain of Ca^{2+} leak function" phenotype of PS1-ΔE9 mutant is consistent with an earlier observation of elevated basal Ca^{2+} levels in the neuronal cells transfected with a PS1-ΔE9 expression construct. Thus, the cells expressing PS1-ΔE9 mutants are expected to be exposed to constitutively elevated cytosolic Ca^{2+} levels, and a partially depleted ER. This contrasts with cells expressing "loss of ER leak function" PS FAD mutants, which are expected to have normal steady-state cytosolic Ca^{2+} levels and an overloaded ER. Interestingly, the PS1-ΔE9 mutation is associated with a unique cotton wool plaque and a spastic paraparesis clinical phenotype (CWP/SP), which is not observed for most other FAD PS1 mutations [310]. It will be very important to determine if other FAD mutations in PS1 associated with the CWP/SP phenotype may also be associated with a "gain of function" for the ER Ca^{2+} leak activity. If such a correlation is established, it would support a causal connection between the ER Ca^{2+} dyshomeostasis and the Aβ pathology in AD.

8.3. Cytoskeletal Pathology in AD and Ca^{2+}

Neurofibrillary tangles, the most overt manifestation of cytoskeletal abnormalities in AD, consist of intracellular fibrillar aggregates of hyperphosphorylated forms of the microtubule-associated protein tau [313]. Tau is normally located in the axons where it maintains microtubules in a polymerized state, but in AD tau dissociates from the microtubules resulting in a microtubule depolymerization and in the accumulation of tau into the cell body. Studies of AD patient brain tissue samples suggest an association between an elevated $[Ca^{2+}]c$ and the neurofibrillary pathology. For example, neurons prone into a neurofibrillary tangle formation are enriched in type II calcium/calmodulin-dependent protein kinase [313], and calpains (Ca^{2+}-dependent proteases that cleave the cytoskeletal proteins) are elevated in vulnerable neuronal populations early in the disease process. Overactivation of glutamate receptors in the hippocampal neurons can cause Ca^{2+}-mediated changes in tau and microtubules similar to those seen in neurofibrillary tangles, suggesting a possible cause-effect relationship between aberrant increases in $(Ca^{2+})c$ and in tangle formation [314]. In addition, Ca^{2+} can cause an AD-like tau phosphorylation and an intracellular Aβ accumulation into the neurons [314]. Conversely, tau mutations that cause a tangle formation in the frontotemporal lobe dementia alter the function of the VACC in a manner that increases the Ca^{2+} influx and may contribute to the cell death process in this disease.

8.4. Ca^{2+} Actions Upstream of the Amyloidogenesis

The placement of the Aβ at the apex of the amyloid cascade hypothesis opposes the fact there must be changes that occur during aging, and AD, that result into an increased production and aggregation of the Aβ. Evidence suggests that Ca^{2+} may be such an upstream factor. Environmental factors that inhibit the amyloidogenesis (caloric restriction, cognitive stimulation and antioxidants) stabilize the neuronal Ca^{2+} homeostasis, whereas factors that enhance the amyloidogenesis disrupt the Ca^{2+} homeostasis. In addition to these kinds of circumstantial evidence, a direct evidence that Ca^{2+} influences APP processing has been reported. Exposure of cultured neurons to Ca^{2+} ionophores increases their production of Aβ, as do conditions such as ischemia that cause sustained elevations of $(Ca^{2+})c$. On the other hand, physiological Ca^{2+} transients (as occur during LTP, for example) increase the α-secretase cleavage of APP and may thereby decrease the Aβ production [310].

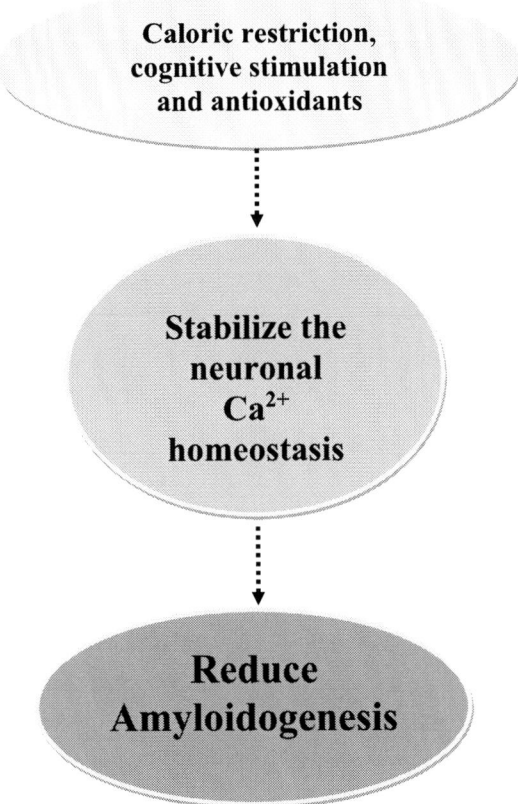

Figure 8.1. Environmental factors that inhibit the amyloidogenesis (caloric restriction, cognitive stimulation and antioxidants) stabilize the neuronal Ca^{2+} homeostasis, whereas factors that enhance the amyloidogenesis disrupt the Ca^{2+} homeostasis.

8.5. Synapses and Ca^{2+}

Studies of patients with a mild cognitive impairment, and AD, suggest that a synaptic dysfunction and degeneration may occur relatively early in the disease process, and studies of AD mouse models uniformly support this tenet. Synaptic terminals are particularly vulnerable to a Ca^{2+}-mediated degeneration because they experience repeated bouts of Ca^{2+} influx and have unusually high energy requirements to support their ion-homeostatic and signalling systems. APP is actively transported to the presynaptic terminals, and considerable evidence suggests that the Aβ is produced and accumulated primarily in the synaptic regions. Aβ can directly disrupt the Ca^{2+} homeostasis in the synaptic terminals by causing a membrane-associated oxidative stress [310]. Consistent with a major role for Aβ in the synaptic damage in AD are data showing a loss of dendritic spines in the dendrites associated with Aβ deposits in APP mutant mice. Aβ also causes a down-regulation of the expression of calcineurin, a Ca^{2+}-activated phosphatase known to play fundamental roles in the synaptic plasticity. Aβ oligomers caused a rapid decrease in the membrane expression of NMDA and EphB2 receptors, followed by an abnormal dendritic spine morphology, and degeneration of spines [310]. The latter effects of Aβ are prevented by a treatment with a NMDA receptor antagonist, suggesting a major role for the Ca^{2+} influx into the dendritic dystrophy. Moreover, an Aβ immunotherapy prevented the synaptic dysfunction, and restores the cognitive function in a mouse model of AD.

Electrophysiological analyses of the synaptic activity in hippocampal slices from APP and PS1 mutant mice have revealed abnormalities in several aspects of Ca^{2+}-mediated synaptic function. APP mutant mice exhibit an abnormal excitatory neuronal activity and a compensatory remodeling of inhibitory circuits in the hippocampus [310]. Expression of the mutant PS1 in cultured hippocampal neurons results in a significant depression of the amplitude of evoked AMPA and NMDA receptor-mediated synaptic currents, and a lower frequency of spontaneous miniature synaptic currents. Aβ impairs a spike-timing-dependent synaptic potentiation at excitatory synapses on neocortical layer 2/3 cortical pyramidal cells in APP mutant mice, which was associated with a decrease in AMPA but not NMDA receptor-mediated currents. Aβ may also perturb the Ca^{2+} handling in neural stem cells resulting into an impaired hippocampal neurogenesis and a compromised ability to form and integrate new neurons from endogenous stem cells.

PS1 mutations have a local adverse effect on synaptic Ca^{2+} regulation that may contribute to a mitochondrial dysfunction and a synaptic degeneration in AD. Thus, synaptosomes from PS1 mutant transgenic mice exhibit enhanced elevations of cytoplasmic Ca^{2+} levels following exposure to depolarizing agents, Aβ, and a mitochondrial toxin compared with synaptosomes from nontransgenic mice, and mice overexpressing wild-type PS1 [310]. Two-photon imaging studies revealed a 10-fold enhancement in the RyR-mediated Ca^{2+} release in spines of PS1-M146V mutant-expressing mice, indicating a major alteration in a synaptic ER Ca^{2+} handling in this AD model. Agents that buffer cytoplasmic Ca^{2+} or that prevent Ca^{2+} release from the ER protected synaptosomes against the adverse effect of PS1 mutations.

Polymorphisms in the apolipoprotein E (ApoE) gene affect one's risk for late onset of AD. Of the three isoforms (E2, E3 and E4), E3 is the most common and E2 the least common. The three isoforms differ at residues 112 and 158; E3 has Cys-112 and Arg-158, whereas E4 has arginine in both positions, and E2 has cysteine in both positions. Inheritance of the allele for E4 isoform is associated with an increased risk and earlier age of the onset of the sporadic AD, whereas E2 reduces the risk [310]. Several studies indicate a potential link between ApoE and the synaptic Ca^{2+} signalling. ApoE2, but not ApoE4, can inhibit an Aβ association with phosphatidylserine in the membrane, providing a potential explanation for the protective effects of ApoE2 in AD. A different line of research demonstrated that the application of low levels of ApoE4 to cultured neurons induces a NMDAR-mediated Ca^{2+} influx and causes a neuronal toxicity. In addition, it was recently demonstrated that reelin can activate the neuronal NMDAR via a src-family tyrosine kinase (SFK)-mediated mechanism, and that reelin association with ApoE receptor 2 (ApoER2) was necessary for an activation of NMDAR. Marked changes in reelin expression levels were observed in brains from both AD patients and AD mouse models, further implicating a potential importance of reelin signalling pathway in AD.

8.6. Selectivity of the Neuronal Vulnerability in AD and Ca^{2+}

Differential production and then deposition of Aβ, resulting into a disruption of Ca^{2+} homeostasis, is one likely determinant of a selective neuronal vulnerability because neurons in brain regions with high Aβ loads (entorhinal cortex, hippocampus, inferior parietal cortex) degenerate, whereas neurons in the regions with little or no Aβ accumulation (cerebellum, striatum, motor cortex) typically do not [315]. However, there are additional factors at work because within a vulnerable brain region (in the presence of similar amounts of Aβ) some neurons degenerate in AD, whereas others do not. Populations of neurons that degenerate in AD typically express high levels of NMDA receptors and have relatively low levels of some Ca^{2+}-binding proteins, compared to resistant neurons [315]. Although hippocampal dentate and CA1 neurons each express NMDA receptors, the dentate neurons express high amounts of calbindin, whereas CA1 neurons do not. Experimental findings suggest that calbindin buffers Ca^{2+} loads and protects neurons against an excitotoxicity; in the hippocampus calbindin-positive neurons are relatively preserved in AD patients with a moderate plaque and tangle content, but in severe cases the calbindin-positive pyramidal cells are also lost, suggesting the possibility that calbindin protects neurons in the early stages of AD. Basal forebrain cholinergic neurons may become depleted of calbindin during aging, which may increase their vulnerability to a degeneration in AD. However, in the entorhinal cortex, calbindin- and parvalbumin-positive non-principal neurons exhibit degenerative changes early in AD, whereas calretinin- and calbindin-positive pyramidal neurons are relatively preserved. Changes in the expression of glutamate receptors may also contribute to an altered neuronal Ca^{2+} handling in AD; as AD progresses, the levels of NR1/2B subunits in hippocampal neurons decrease, while the NR2A subunit levels remain unchanged.

Other factors that may contribute to a selective neuronal vulnerability in AD by perturbing the Ca^{2+} homeostasis are neuron-specific differences in energy metabolism, antioxidant systems and a neurotrophic factor support [315].

8.7. IMPROVING NEURONAL CA^{2+} HOMEOSTASIS AS A THERAPEUTIC APPROACH FOR AD

Because aging is the major risk factor for AD and other neurodegenerative diseases, it follows that interventions that counteract the aging process would protect neurons against excessive Ca^{2+}, and AD. Epidemiological and experimental evidence suggests that exercise, dietary energy restriction and the cognitive stimulation may retard the aging processes and protect against AD. Indeed, environmental enrichment, exercise and dietary energy restriction suppress the disease process, and enhance the cognitive performance in mouse models of AD. These beneficial environmental factors may act, in part, by inducing the expression of neurotrophic factors such as BDNF, that stabilize the neuronal Ca^{2+} homeostasis. Antioxidants and cellular energy-promoting agents might also be expected to stabilize the neuronal Ca^{2+} homeostasis and to protect against AD. Because an increased Aβ production, and accumulation, at synapses is of major importance in AD pathogenesis, treatments that reduce the Aβ production or enhance its clearance from the brain are being vigorously pursued. One of the most promising anti-Aβ approaches that is currently being tested in patients is immunization with Aβ or treatment with purified Aβ antibodies. By removing Aβ from the brain, immunization would be expected to prevent or reverse the Aβ-induced neuronal Ca^{2+} dysregulation.

Table 8.1. The Ca²⁺/cAMP signalling dysregulations and their consequences

Disruption of Ca²⁺/cAMP signalling			
↑ [Ca²⁺]c		↓ [cAMP]c	
Abnormal cellular consequences			
Increase of the neuronal death	Increase of the catecholamines' release	Neuroinflammation	Increase of β-cell apoptosis and decrease of the insulin levels
Symptoms and clinical consequences			
Neurodegeneration and neuroinflammation	Sympathetic hyperactivity	Dysregulation of transmitter release (e.g., monoamines)	Dysregulations of the glucose homeostasis and stimulation of inflammatory processes
Disorders			
Dementia	Hypertension	Depression	Diabetes

Symbols - Up arrow: increasing; Down arrow: decreasing; (Ca²⁺)c: intracellular concentration of Ca²⁺; (cAMP)c: intracellular concentration of cAMP.

8.8. REASONABLE MECHANISMS FOR HEALTHY BRAIN AGING AND AD

Healthy brain aging can be promoted by regular exercise, moderation in caloric intake and engaging in intellectually challenging activities. These lifestyle factors may stabilize the neuronal Ca²⁺ homeostasis. Drugs that inhibit β- or γ-secretases are another viable approach for reducing the Aβ production and an associated Ca²⁺-mediated neurotoxicity. Drugs that target specific Ca²⁺-regulating systems (downstream of age- and Aβ-related disruption of Ca^{2+} homeostasis) provide another approach. Indeed, the only drug thus far shown to slow the disease progression in AD patients is the NMDA receptor open channel blocker memantine, as described above. Beneficial effects have also been reported in AD clinical trials of Dimebon, a drug that has been claimed to stabilize the Ca^{2+} signalling by blocking the NMDAR and voltage-activated Ca^{2+} channels. As with other major age-related diseases (cardiovascular disease, diabetes and cancers), a risk reduction for AD may be achievable by a dietary moderation, and exercise, combined with dietary supplements (omega-3 fatty acids and folic acid, for example). For individuals at high risk for AD (ApoE4 genotype and family history, for example), prophylactic approaches may be prescribed, including anti-inflammatory drugs and an immunization (see Table 8.1).

Chapter 9

HYPERTENSION AND HIGHER RISK FOR THE DECLINE OF COGNITION

Epidemiological and clinical studies have been reporting a clinical link between hypertension and higher risk for decline of cognition, such as that observed in AD patients [316]. However, the clinical link between hypertension and the development of AD is not fully elucidated. Could this link be just a forged association?

In fact, no! Hypertension, mostly midlife high blood pressure, has been clearly linked with an increased risk for cognitive decline [316, 317]. Some reports have been showing an increased incidence of neurodegenerative diseases, like AD, in people with high blood pressure [316-318]. In addition, with aging comes higher incidence of atherosclerosis, which is a predictive issue for high blood pressure in later life. Thus, atherosclerosis, as well as sustained hypertension, may induce cerebral ischemia and hypoxia in senile people. Then, these issues may worsen cognitive function. Furthermore, midlife hypertension (age 40-64 years) increases the incidence of AD in later life (≥65 years); and hypertension has been linked with increased amyloid deposition and neurofibrillary tangles, both hallmarks of AD [319]. Indeed, compared to the brains of normotensive patients, the brains of patients with a history of hypertension show greater levels of β-amyloid plaques (Aβ), atrophy and neurofibrillary tangles [320, 321]. Thus, hypertension has been recognized as a risk issue for cortical fibrillar β-amyloid deposits, and also lower glucose metabolism in some AD brain regions [322].

In addition, observational and epidemiological reports have been showing that antihypertensive therapy could have neuroprotective effects on cognitive impairment originated from neurodegenerative diseases [323]. Some reports showed that CCBs would be the most advantageous: they could decrease the risk for, and progression of, cognitive impairment by lowering blood pressure, and through a neuroprotective specific effect [324].

It is evidenced that certain CCBs, such as dihydropyridine, which are more effective at crossing the blood brain barrier, present some pleiotropic effects such as reducing Aβ production, and stimulating Aβ clearance, across the blood brain barrier [320]. Whether the effects showed in cell culture, and in animal models, translate into humans deserves more attention. According to the Syst-Eur Trial, a CCB entitled nitrendipine, compared with placebo, decreased the risk of neurodegenerative diseases by 55%. This Syst-Eur Trial is the most significant randomized control trial of hypertension to have evidenced statistically significant positive effects of nitrendipine to decrease the incidence of AD [325]. It is interesting to highlight that the diuretic thiazide, chlortalidone, did not protect against cognitive impairment, while reduction of blood pressure was comparable in the Syst-Eur Trial, suggesting that nitrendipine has a neuroprotective effect beyond its property to reduce blood pressure [325, 326]. Intriguingly, a retrospective population-based cohort report, involving thousands of senile hypertensive patients, demonstrated that prescription of CCBs reduced the risk of neurodegenerative diseases like AD, indicating that these pharmaceuticals could be clinically used to treat neurodegenerative diseases [6]. Thus, which is (are) the virtual mechanism(s) of action for the CCBs pleiotropic effects?

As described above, amyloid plaques, a histological hallmark of AD, are comprised of extracellular aggregates of the amyloid beta, Aβ, which is believed to be a pivotal mediator of neuronal degeneration, and impaired cognitive function in AD [319]. Aβ has been linked, for example, with elevated $(Ca^{2+})_c$, and increased vulnerability of the neurons to excitotoxicity [319]. Then, a virtual mechanism of action for CCBs neuroprotective effects could be attributed to a restoration and maintenance of Ca^{2+} homeostasis, which is dysregulated in the neurodegenerative diseases, due to a reduction of neuronal Ca^{2+} influx. The possible role of the Ca^{2+}/cAMP signalling interaction in these CCBs pleiotropic effects, including the possible role of the Ca^{2+}/cAMP signalling interaction in the association between hypertension and higher risk for the decline of cognition, should also be considered.

Chapter 10

HYPERTENSION AND HIGHER RISK FOR DIABETES

Hypertensive patients present a higher risk for diabetes [327], considered a classical predictive issue for cardiovascular diseases. In addition, diabetes and hypertension frequently occur together. Indeed, concerning the diseases´ mechanisms, there is substantial interaction between diabetes and hypertension [328]. Furthermore, obesity, inflammation, oxidative stress and insulin resistance may be considered to be the upstream issues for these diseases. Recent advances in the understanding of how combating these issues have provided new insights and perspectives for the treatment of both diseases. For instance, the scientific literature classically considers physical activity as an important protective role for these two diseases. Thus, understanding the diseases´ mechanisms, and their interactions, may allow a more effective and proactive therapeutic approach for their prevention and treatment [327, 328].

Concerning epidemiological aspects, hypertension and diabetes are considered two of the leading risk issues for atherosclerosis and its associated side effects, including heart attacks and strokes. In the Hong Kong Cardiovascular Risk Factor Prevalence Study, just 42% of patients with diabetes had normal blood pressure, and only 56% of patients with hypertension had normal glucose tolerance [329]. In the United States, hypertension is presented in approximately 50% to 80% in patients with type 2 diabetes [330]. In addition, a prospective cohort study in the United States demonstrated that hypertensive patients had an increased risk of almost 2.5 times to develop type 2 diabetes, compared to normotensive patients [331]. In fact, diabetes and hypertension are presented in the same individual more often than would occur by causality, whereas the interaction between dysglycemia and raised blood pressure is even more significant [332]. Then, suggesting both common genetic or environmental issues in their etiology [329].

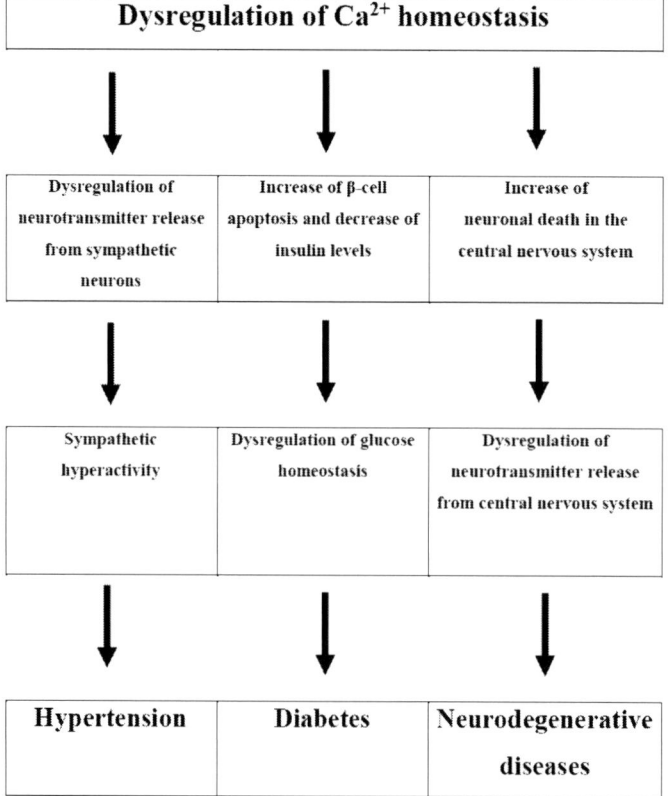

Figure 8.2. The Ca^{2+} homeostasis dysregulation and its endpoint consequences: hypertension, diabetes and neurodegenerative diseases.

About therapeutics for diabetes, in patients treated with CCBs, it can be observed an improvement of diabetes status such as glycemic control [333]. The virtual mechanisms of action remain under discussion. Indeed, leaving from epidemiological aspects and going into cellular mechanisms, the decline of β-cell function is a classical hallmark of diabetes, but there are no current treatment approaches that could successfully restore this decline. Xu et al [334]. Discovered that CCBs can enhance endogenous insulin levels, and rescue mice from STZ-induced diabetes. These authors also found that CCBs promoted β-cell survival and improved glucose homeostasis, including insulin sensitivity in BTBR ob/ob mice. The authors concluded that these CCBs pleiotropic effects could be partially mediated due to a reduction of intracellular Ca^{2+} [334]. The possible role of the Ca^{2+}/cAMP signalling interaction in these CCBs pleiotropic effects, including the possible role of the Ca^{2+}/cAMP signalling interaction in the association between hypertension and higher risk for diabetes, should also be considered. The Figure 8.2 summarizes the previous discussion.

Chapter 11

A LINK BETWEEN DIABETES AND DEMENTIA

In the last years, the relationship between diabetes and memory dysfunctions has been explored [335-338]. It was shown that T2DM has been correlated to a decreasing in both psychomotor speed and processing, including a memory deficit related to speech, instant and late recall, visual retaining and attention, and verbal fluency [335-338]. In addition, diabetes patients demonstrated both a lack of balance and increased falls, including slower walking speed, but it is still unclear if the influence of diabetes on the cerebral functionality could subsidize the rising of these symptoms [335-338].

Furthermore, it was also observed that cardiovascular diseases increase the risk of presenting dementia [339]. In fact, subclinical cardiovascular and atherosclerosis markers, in addition to stroke, are correlated to a decreasing of cognitive abilities in T2DM patients [340]. Indeed, mild cognitive impairment was observed in ~ 42% of these diabetic patients [340]. In another report, the link between diabetes and a cognitive imbalance was also examined, concluding that patients with T2DM showed a lower score in the Mini-Mental State Examination (than those without diabetes) [341]. Another study [19] evaluated whether lesions in the brain related to both vascular and degenerative issues could underlie the correlation between diabetes and a reduced cognitive performance, including to which magnitude [342]. It was also concluded that diabetes patients' speed of executing functions and processing, in addition to memory performance, was significantly reduced compared to the control group [342].

In fact, reports involving neuroimaging and neuropathological issues have also endorsed that diabetes plays a role in neurodegeneration [343]. For instance, brain atrophy was concluded to be highly correlated to T2DM [343], which usually progresses up to 3 times quicker, compared to the physiological aging [21, 22]. T2DM patients also demonstrated an enhanced incidence of dementia, like Alzheimer's disease (AD) [344, 345], and also an increased incidence of vascular dementia. Finally, about 17.5% of patients with T2DM have demonstrated from a moderate to a severe deficiency in daily activities [346, 347], whereas 11.3% have demonstrated an impairment of cognitive functions, and 14.2% have demonstrated signs of depression [348], thus negatively influencing the cognitive functions and daily activities [348].

In fact, a lower brain glucose metabolism, a clinical sign of diabetes, is presented even before the onset of a measurable cognitive decline in two groups of patients at risk of AD: in those patients who express the apolipoprotein E4 and in those with a maternal family history of AD [349]. Several evidences from *in vitro* and animal studies suggest that a brain glucose hypometabolism may precede and, therefore, may contribute to the neuropathologic cascade, resulting in a cognitive decline in AD [349]. The explanation for why brain glucose hypometabolism develops is uncertain, but may include: defects in brain glucose transport, a disrupted glycolysis and/or an impaired mitochondrial function. In addition, aging is correlated to an increased risk of deteriorating the systemic control of glucose utilization, which, in turn, may enhance the risk of declining brain glucose uptake, at least in some brain regions [349, 350]. Then, therapeutic strategies to reduce the risk of AD could include: 1) enhancing insulin sensitivity by improving systemic glucose utilization or (2) circumventing deterioration of brain glucose metabolism by using approaches that safely induce sustainable ketonemia [350].

Moreover, considering there are common inflammatory pathways involved in both AD and T2DM, the neuronal dysfunction related to dementia may include the disruption of several biochemical pathways, and one of them has been suggested to be linked to the tyrosine hydroxylase (TH) [351]. It has been argued that TH is affected by the β-amyloid protein, then providing a link between dementia and TH loss.

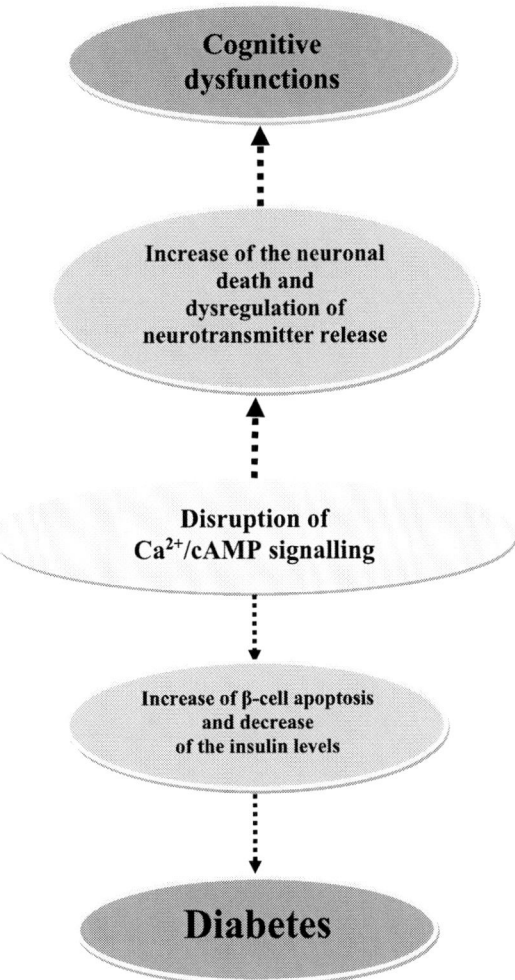

Figure 8.3. Disruption of Ca^{2+}/cAMP signalling and its consequences.

Besides inducing sustainable ketonemia, additional therapeutic strategies to treat both AD and T2DM may result from plants which have constituents related to antiaging properties (due to the presence of antioxidants) [352]. In fact, many plants have high medicinal properties to be explored. However, determining the components that have a specific pharmacological activity, and their clinical effects, still remains a challenge. For instance, an interesting issue compiled 10 intriguing reports focusing on medicinal plants with the potential for the management of both diabetes and neurodegenerative diseases [352]. Considering that AD is a systemic process, involving multiple pathophysiological issues, a combination of pharmacotherapy and nonpharmacological interventions has been proposed to treat dementia. The nonpharmacological interventions also include increasing the sensory input through physical and mental activities with the aim of modifying the cerebral blood flow, in addition to implementing nutritional interventions such as diet modification and vitamins, besides nutraceuticals therapy for vitalizing brain functioning.

The previous discussion has been summarized in the Figure 8.3.

Chapter 12

SYNOPSIS

The diagnosis of neurological and psychiatric disorders, especially the neurodegenerative diseases like Parkinson's and Alzheimer's diseases relies critically on the clinical diagnosis of patients. In addition, emerging therapies may supplement a clinical assessment in the next years. Although the pharmacological therapies have been largely unsuccessful in attenuating neurodegenerative diseases symptoms, targeting potential risk factors aiming to decrease the incidence of these neurodegenerative diseases is an important public health issue. Finally, novel strategies to treat these diseases, throughout our recent discovery entitled *"calcium paradox"* phenomenon due to the Ca^{2+}/cAMP interaction could greatly contribute to enhance pharmacological therapeutic strategies for increasing a neuroprotection and enhancing the neurotransmission, including Alzheimer's and Parkinson's diseases, and depression. As in the diseases like Alzheimer's and Parkinson's, this pharmacological strategy could be used to increase the neurotransmission, and neuroprotection, in the neurodegenerative diseases like the amyotrophic lateral sclerosis and myasthenia gravis. For instance, considering a $(Ca^{2+})c$ elevation could contribute to both: negatively to the neuroprotective effects and positively to the exocytosis, it may be promising the therapeutic use of the PDE inhibitors in combination with the CCB for antidepressant and neuroprotective purposes [14]. By reducing the Ca^{2+}

influx, the CCB may increase (cAMP)c by enhancing the AC activity, which increases the neuroprotection. cAMP also enhances the release of Ca^{2+} from the ER, which increases the exocytosis in the secretory cells [6]. Thus, we have in this scenario the following targets for medicines: AC, PDE, L-type VACC, PKA and RyR/IP$_3$R. In conclusion, the association of typical psychiatric/neurological medicines with the CCB or PDE inhibitor rolipram could dramatically improve the psychiatric and neurological therapies, mainly by reducing the adverse effects and improving effectiveness of these current medicines.

In the field of drug interaction, we could also infer that a therapy involving the combination of drugs which increase (cAMP)c, like rolipram, with low doses of the CCB like verapamil should be done carefully in hypertensive patients with neurological/psychiatric disorders, considering the role of the sympathetic transmission in regulating the vascular tone by releasing neurotransmitters into the vasculature. For example, patients both psychiatrically depressed and hypertensive taking drugs which increase (cAMP)c, concomitantly with the CCB, may worsen their hypertensive status, even though ameliorating their depression. In addition, a combination of the L-type CCB and rolipram could be used to enhance the neurotransmission and mitigate a deleterious excess of Ca^{2+} influx, a condition seen in aging and in the neurodegenerative diseases [250]. These hypotheses need further investigation in experiments with animal models of disease as well as in clinical trials.

Chapter 13

FUTURE DIRECTIONS

The solution for the so-called "calcium paradox" has been revealed 4 years ago, when we demonstrated the involvement of the interaction between Ca^{2+} and cAMP signalling pathways (Ca^{2+}/cAMP signalling interaction) in this enigma. The "calcium paradox" emerged 4 decades ago, when numerous clinical studies have concluded that the prescription of the L-type Ca^{2+} channel blockers (CCBs) for hypertensive patients decreased the arterial pressure but produced a stimulation of sympathetic hyperactivity. Indeed, initially these adverse effects of the CCBs have been attributed to the adjust reflex of arterial pressure, but this conclusion remained not completely satisfactory. The year of 2013 would change this history forever! Through an original experiment, we revealed that the "calcium paradox" phenomenon came from an increased transmitter release from the sympathetic neurons stimulated by the CCBs due to their handling on the Ca^{2+}/cAMP signalling interaction. It is now well-established that the signalling pathways mediated by Ca^{2+} and cAMP can interact, thus playing a vital role in the cellular processes of mammalians. In clinical pharmacology, it has opened novel opportunities for the development of pharmaceuticals more efficient, and safer, for treating neurodegenerative diseases. Then, the manipulation of the Ca^{2+}/cAMP signalling interaction could improve therapeutic strategies for stimulating the synaptic transmission compromised by a transmitter release deficit and attenuating the death of neurons. More recently, the manipulation of this interaction has been proposed by us to inhibit the cancer progression, another interesting avenue for medical research.

In fact, it was shown that the prescription of the L-type CCBs can reduce the motor symptoms and reduces the continued neuronal death in the animal model of Parkinson's disease, indicating that the L-type CCBs are potentially workable neuroprotective pharmaceuticals. Intriguingly, a 1-decade study involving thousands of senile hypertensive patients demonstrated that the prescription of L-type CCBs can reduce the blood pressure, and the incidence of dementia in hypertensive patients, indicating that these pharmaceuticals could be used to treat the neurodegenerative diseases in clinics. These results for the effects related to a neuroprotection of the CCBs have been reinvestigated in thousands of elderly hypertensive patients with a dysfunction of memory abilities. These studies concluded that the patients who have taken CCBs had their risk of cognitive dysfunction decreased, such as Alzheimer's disease. These findings reinforce the concept that the L-type CCBs can reduce a cytosolic Ca^{2+} overload produced due to a blocking of Ca^{2+} influx, and thus could be an alternative pharmacological goal to reduce, or to prevent, death of neurons resulting from neurodegenerative diseases.

Based on these findings, we have anticipated that the pharmacological regulation of the Ca^{2+}/cAMP signalling interaction by the combined use of the L-type CCBs and (cAMP)c-enhancer compounds could be a novel therapeutic goal for increasing the neurotransmission in neurological and psychiatric disorders resulting from a neurotransmitter release deficit and neuronal death. This pharmacological strategy opens a novel pathway for the drug development more efficient for the treatment of Alzheimer's and other neurodegenerative diseases.

In addition, it has been shown that the dysregulation of intracellular signalling pathways mediated by Ca^{2+} and cAMP participates in the cancer initiation, tumor formation, tumor progression, metastasis, invasion and angiogenesis. Thereby, proteins involved in these pathways, such as the Ca^{2+} channels and cAMP-dependent protein kinase (PKA), represent potential drug targets for the cancer therapy [353-359]. With this concept in mind, some studies showed that drugs able to interfere with the intracellular Ca^{2+} signalling such as selective CCBs, as amlodipine, inhibit proliferative response in different cancer cells. In addition, drugs able to increase the intracellular cAMP levels (cAMP-enhancer compounds), such as phosphodiesterase (PDE) 4 inhibitors, have been proposed as potential adjuvant, chemotherapeutic or chemopreventive agents in some cancer types, including the hepatocellular carcinoma. Then, the pharmacological modulation of the intracellular signalling mediated by Ca^{2+} and cAMP in the cancer cells may represent a new therapeutic strategy for the cancer progression.

Chapter 14

CONCLUSION

"Science is not always linear! Imagine this scenario: the PhD researcher and his supervisor are formulating their experiment. During the experiment course, there is on the bench a residual solution containing Verapamil, a L-type Ca^{2+} channel blocker (CCB). In a relapse, the PhD researcher decides to add this solution in an isolated smooth muscle preparation. The smooth muscle was prior relaxed with a drug that increased the cAMP cytosolic concentration. According to the classical receptor theory, addition of verapamil in the smooth muscle preparation should enhance the relaxation of the smooth muscle! To his surprise, the PhD researcher observed an incredible contraction of the smooth muscle! Perplexed with this result, the PhD researcher and his supervisor did not know how to explain this phenomenon immediately."

Indeed, the previous described scenario happened during my PhD studies performed in the laboratory of Prof. Afonso Caricati-Neto at EPM-UNIFESP. According to the classical concepts of neurotransmission described since Sir Henry Dale, the release of neurotransmitters critically depends on the Ca^{2+} influx through L-type voltage-activated Ca^{2+} channels (VACCs), thus culminating in the elevation of Ca^{2+} concentration $(Ca^{2+})c$. As a consequence, this increases the release of the neurotransmitter, finally enhancing the contraction of the smooth muscle. Considering these concepts, some authors showed that verapamil reduced the contraction of the smooth muscles. Nonetheless, science is not always linear! Surprisingly, a study published in the 1970's described that, besides the classical effect of verapamil (in high concentrations) to reduce the smooth muscle contractions, verapamil could also produce an apparent paradoxical increase of those contractions (in low concentrations). Isn't it strange, puzzling, a "calcium paradox"? This apparent puzzling result was validated in 1981 by French and Scott. Additionally, another study described that verapamil augmented the smooth muscle contractions, whose effect was replicated by diltiazem (another L-type VACC blocker). The authors concluded that this result could be attributed to an agonist effect of verapamil on the L-type VACCs! Really?! Years later, another outstanding study appeared revealing that the L- type VACCs blocker (verapamil) elicited similar increases of the contractions of the smooth muscle; the authors did not provide an elucidation for such apparent paradoxical observation. No one could blame on them!

Since 1990's, the Prof. Afonso's lab. has also reproduced those previous observations: at lower concentrations, the CCB produced a slight increase, while at higher concentrations the VACCs blocker caused a decrease of the smooth muscle contractions. In 2013, during my PhD studies, we found an exciting discovery: as the high verapamil concentrations, various cAMP-stimulating compounds classically relax the isolated smooth muscle. Surprisingly, in the presence of cAMP-stimulating compounds, the lower concentrations of verapamil caused an extraordinary augmentation of the smooth muscle contractions, instead of inhibiting them! In a "eureka minute," we concluded that the interaction between Ca^{2+} and cAMP signalling pathways (Ca^{2+}/cAMP signalling interaction) could properly solve these paradoxical results, including those observed since 1970's. The original paper published by us in Cell Calcium (2013) has appeared four times in ScienceDirect TOP 25 Hottest Articles lists, including the TOP 1 positions.

Which is the relevance of this discovery for the neurodegenerative diseases? The rising increment in the life expectancy of the world's population has increased the fear about the age-related neurodegenerative disorders, such as Alzheimer's (AD) and Parkinson's (PD) diseases, and others. It is now well recognized that an imbalance of intracellular Ca^{2+} homeostasis contributes to the pathogenesis of neurological diseases such as the neurodegenerative diseases, including AD and PD, among others. Our discovery of the role of the Ca^{2+}/cAMP signalling interaction in the neurotransmission, and neuroprotection, has subsidized the understanding of the pathophysiology, and pharmacology, of the neurological and psychiatric diseases, opening a large pathway for the advancement of new pharmacological strategies (more effective) for the treatment of these disorders. In 2013, as described above, we discovered that the "calcium paradox" resulted from an increase of transmitter release from the sympathetic neurons stimulated by CCB due to their modulatory action on the Ca^{2+}/cAMP signalling interaction. In addition, we discovered that this modulatory action of the CCBs both increases the intracellular levels of cAMP and reduces the Ca^{2+} influx, thus attenuating the neuronal death in the neurodegenerative diseases resulted from a cytosolic Ca^{2+} excess. This novel proposal involves pharmaceuticals already approved, and clinically safe, from non-neurodegenerative therapy indications. These concepts have been extensively discussed in several cited international articles of my own authorship (> 60), book chapters and in an international book.

The prescription of the L-type CCBs in hypertensive patients has been reported to decrease the arterial pressure, but also produces a sympathetic hyperactivity. Initially, these adverse effects of the CCBs have been attributed to the adjust reflex of arterial pressure, but this conclusion remained not completely satisfactory. The year of 2013 would change this history forever! Through a creative experiment, we revealed that the solution for this so-called "calcium paradox" phenomenon was due to an increase of the transmitter release from the sympathetic neurons achieved by CCBs due to their handling on the interaction between Ca^{2+} and cAMP signalling pathways. We demonstrated that the contractions of the smooth muscle (vas deferens) were completely inhibited by the L-type CCBs in high concentrations (>1 µmol/L), but puzzlingly increased in concentrations below 1 µmol/L, thus defined as a sympathetic hyperactivity promoted by CCBs. Our studies clearly established that the contradictory sympathetic hyperactivity is due to an augmentation of the transmitter release from sympathetic neurons achieved by L-type CCBs due to their interference on the interaction between Ca^{2+} and cAMP signalling pathways. In fact, many reports have shown that an elevation of cytosolic cAMP concentration ((cAMP)c) reduces the neuronal death resulted from a cytosolic Ca^{2+} overload, then stimulating a neuroprotective effect. As mentioned above, the L-type CCBs increase the transmitter release due to their handling on the interaction between Ca^{2+} and cAMP signalling pathways. This interference activates the ACs, causing an elevation of (cAMP)c that, in turn, induces a Ca^{2+} release from the ER that stimulates the transmitter release. In addition, this elevation of (cAMP)c produces neuroprotective effects mediated by the Ca^{2+} and cAMP signalling pathways. It was proposed that this neuroprotective effect results from an activation by cAMP on the cellular survival pathways mediated by PKA/CREB. Then, the pharmacological interference of the Ca^{2+}/cAMP signalling interaction from the combined use of the L-type CCBs prescribed in the antihypertensive therapy, and (cAMP)c-enhancer compounds prescribed in the anti-depressive therapy like rolipram, could be a novel pharmacological goal for increasing the neurotransmission in neurological and psychiatric disorders resulted from a deficit of the neurotransmitter release, and neuronal death.

In conclusion, pharmacological interference on the interaction between Ca^{2+} and cAMP signalling pathways could be a more efficient therapeutic approach for enhancing the neurotransmission resulted from a neurotransmitter release deficit and reducing the neuronal death in the neurodegenerative diseases (like Alzheimer's and Parkinson's diseases). More recently, the manipulation of this interaction has been proposed by us to inhibit the cancer progression, another avenue for medical research. These findings could dramatically impact in the clinical pharmacology [320-322].

BIBLIOGRAPHY

[1] Grossman E, Messerli FH. Effect of calcium antagonists on sympathetic activity. *European heart journal*. 1998;19 Suppl F:F27-31.

[2] Koslov DS, Andersson KE. Physiological and pharmacological aspects of the vas deferens-an update. *Frontiers in pharmacology*. 4:101.

[3] Bomfim GH, Verde LF, Frussa-Filho R, Jurkiewicz A, Jurkiewicz NH. Functional effects of alcohol withdrawal syndrome on peripheral sympathetic neurotransmission in vas deferens of adult rats. *Life sciences*. 108(1):34-43.

[4] Caricati-Neto A, D'Angelo L C, Reuter H, Hyppolito Jurkiewicz N, Garcia AG, Jurkiewicz A. Enhancement of purinergic neurotransmission by galantamine and other acetylcholinesterase inhibitors in the rat vas deferens. *European journal of pharmacology*. 2004;503(1-3):191-201.

[5] Burnstock G, Fredholm BB, North RA, Verkhratsky A. The birth and postnatal development of purinergic signalling. *Acta physiologica* (Oxford, England).199(2):93-147.

[6] Bergantin LB, Souza CF, Ferreira RM, Smaili SS, Jurkiewicz NH, Caricati-Neto A, et al. Novel model for "calcium paradox" in sympathetic transmission of smooth muscles: role of cyclic AMP pathway. *Cell Calcium*. 2013;54(3):202-12.

[7] Burnstock G. Autonomic neurotransmission: 60 years since sir Henry Dale. *Annu Rev Pharmacol Toxicol*. 2009;49:1-30.

[8] Hidalgo A, Beneit J, Lorenzo P. (Effect of calcium antagonists on the response of the rat vas deferens to noradrenaline and field stimulation). *Rev Esp Fisiol*. 1983;39(2):211-5.

[9] Hata F, Fujita A, Saeki K, Kishi I, Takeuchi T, Yagasaki O. Selective inhibitory effects of calcium channel antagonists on the two components of the neurogenic response of guinea pig vas deferens. *J Pharmacol Exp Ther*. 1992;263(1):214-20.

[10] Kreye VA, Luth JB. Proceedings: Verapamil-induced phasic contractions of the isolated rat vas deferens. Naunyn Schmiedebergs *Arch Pharmacol*. 1975;287 Suppl:R43.

[11] French AM, Scott NC. A comparison of the effects of nifedipine and verapamil on rat vas deferens. *Br J Pharmacol*. 1981;73(2):321-3.

[12] Moritoki H, Iwamoto T, Kanaya J, Maeshiba Y, Ishida Y, Fukuda H. Verapamil enhances the non-adrenergic twitch response of rat vas deferens. *Eur J Pharmacol*. 1987;140(1):75-83.

[13] Rae GA, Calixto JB. Interactions of calcium antagonists and the calcium channel agonist Bay K 8644 on neurotransmission of the mouse isolated vas deferens. *Br J Pharmacol*. 1989;96(2):333-40.

[14] Caricati-Neto A, Garcia AG, Bergantin LB. Pharmacological implications of the $Ca^{(2+)}$/cAMP signaling interaction: from risk for antihypertensive therapy to potential beneficial for neurological and psychiatric disorders. *Pharmacol Res Perspect*. 2015;3(5):e00181.

[15] Bergantin LB, Jurkiewicz A, García AG, Caricati-Neto A. A calcium paradox in the context of neurotransmission. *Journal of Pharmacy and Pharmacology*. 2015;3:9.

[16] Rang HP. The receptor concept: pharmacology's big idea. *British journal of pharmacology*. 2006;147 Suppl 1:S9-16.

[17] Roberts OL, Dart C. cAMP signalling in the vasculature: the role of Epac (exchange protein directly activated by cAMP). *Biochemical Society transactions.* 42(1):89-97.

[18] Marcantoni A, Carabelli V, Vandael DH, Comunanza V, Carbone E. PDE type-4 inhibition increases L-type $Ca^{(2+)}$ currents, action potential firing, and quantal size of exocytosis in mouse chromaffin cells. *Pflugers Arch.* 2009;457(5):1093-110.

[19] Pirisino R, Banchelli G, Ignesti G, Mantelli L, Matucci R, Raimondi L, et al. Calcium modulatory properties of 2,6-dibutylbenzylamine (B25) in rat isolated vas deferens, cardiac and smooth muscle preparations. *Br J Pharmacol.* 1993;109(4):1038-45.

[20] Rosa JM, Conde M, Nanclares C, Orozco A, Colmena I, de Pascual R, et al. Paradoxical facilitation of exocytosis by inhibition of L-type calcium channels of bovine chromaffin cells. *Biochem Biophys Res Commun.* 2011;410(2):307-11.

[21] Fontaine J, Lebrun P. Pharmacological analysis of the effects of Bay K 8644 and organic calcium antagonists on the mouse isolated distal colon. *Br J Pharmacol.* 1988;94(4):1198-205.

[22] Garcia AG, Sala F, Reig JA, Viniegra S, Frias J, Fonteriz R, et al. Dihydropyridine BAY-K-8644 activates chromaffin cell calcium channels. *Nature.* 1984;309(5963):69-71.

[23] Ahuja M, Jha A, Maleth J, Park S, Muallem S. cAMP and Ca signaling in secretory epithelia: Crosstalk and synergism. *Cell Calcium.* 2014.

[24] Nishimura M, Asai F, Urakawa N. Verapamil-induced transmitter release in rat diaphragm muscle. *Jpn J Pharmacol.* 1982;32(2):231-5.

[25] Koshi T. (Abnormal secretory response to verapamil of pancreatic B cells of neonatal rats maintained in high glucose). *Nihon Naibunpi Gakkai Zasshi.* 1993;69(9):973-88.

[26] Rosa JM, de Diego AM, Gandia L, Garcia AG. L-type calcium channels are preferentially coupled to endocytosis in bovine chromaffin cells. *Biochem Biophys Res Commun.* 2007;357(4):834-9.

[27] Rosa JM, Gandia L, Garcia AG. Inhibition of N and PQ calcium channels by calcium entry through L channels in chromaffin cells. *Pflugers Arch.* 2009;458(4):795-807.

[28] Lopez MG, Villarroya M, Lara B, Martinez Sierra R, Albillos A, Garcia AG, et al. Q- and L-type Ca^{2+} channels dominate the control of secretion in bovine chromaffin cells. *FEBS Lett.* 1994;349(3):331-7.

[29] Xiong W, Liu T, Wang Y, Chen X, Sun L, Guo N, et al. An inhibitory effect of extracellular Ca^{2+} on Ca^{2+}-dependent exocytosis. *PloS one.* 6(10):e24573.

[30] Shang S, Wang C, Liu B, Wu Q, Zhang Q, Liu W, et al. Extracellular Caper se inhibits quantal size of catecholamine release in adrenal slice chromaffin cells. *Cell calcium.*

[31] Bruce JI, Shuttleworth TJ, Giovannucci DR, Yule DI. Phosphorylation of inositol 1,4,5-trisphosphate receptors in parotid acinar cells. A mechanism for the synergistic effects of cAMP on Ca^{2+} signaling. *J Biol Chem.* 2002;277(2):1340-8.

[32] Chatton JY, Cao Y, Liu H, Stucki JW. Permissive role of cAMP in the oscillatory Ca^{2+} response to inositol 1,4,5-trisphosphate in rat hepatocytes. *Biochem J.* 1998;330 (Pt 3):1411-6.

[33] Lee RJ, Foskett JK. cAMP-activated Ca^{2+} signaling is required for CFTR-mediated serous cell fluid secretion in porcine and human airways. *J Clin Invest.* 2010;120(9):3137-48.

[34] Fechner L, Baumann O, Walz B. Activation of the cyclic AMP pathway promotes serotonin-induced Ca^{2+} oscillations in salivary glands of the blowfly *Calliphora vicina*. *Cell Calcium.* 2013;53(2):94-101.

[35] Wu PC, Fann MJ, Kao LS. Characterization of Ca^{2+} signaling pathways in mouse adrenal medullary chromaffin cells. *Journal of neurochemistry.* 112(5):1210-22.

[36] Morita K, Dohi T, Kitayama S, Koyama Y, Tsujimoto A. Enhancement of stimulation-evoked catecholamine release from cultured bovine adrenal chromaffin cells by forskolin. *Journal of neurochemistry.* 1987;48(1):243-7.

[37] Fleckenstein A. History of calcium antagonists. *Circ Res.* 1983;52(2 Pt 2):I3-16.

[38] Garcia AG, Garcia-De-Diego AM, Gandia L, Borges R, Garcia-Sancho J. Calcium signaling and exocytosis in adrenal chromaffin cells. *Physiol Rev.* 2006;86(4):1093-131.

[39] Morita K, Dohi T, Kitayama S, Koyama Y, Tsujimoto A. Stimulation-evoked Ca^{2+} fluxes in cultured bovine adrenal chromaffin cells are enhanced by forskolin. *Journal of neurochemistry.* 1987;48(1):248-52.

[40] Anderson K, Robinson PJ, Marley PD. Cholinoceptor regulation of cyclic AMP levels in bovine adrenal medullary cells. *Br J Pharmacol.* 1992;106(2):360-6.

[41] Przywara DA, Guo X, Angelilli ML, Wakade TD, Wakade AR. A non-cholinergic transmitter, pituitary adenylate cyclase-activating polypeptide, utilizes a novel mechanism to evoke catecholamine secretion in rat adrenal chromaffin cells. *J Biol Chem.* 1996;271(18):10545-50.

[42] Marley PD. Mechanisms in histamine-mediated secretion from adrenal chromaffin cells. *Pharmacol Ther.* 2003;98(1):1-34.

[43] Wilson SP. Vasoactive intestinal peptide elevates cyclic AMP levels and potentiates secretion in bovine adrenal chromaffin cells. *Neuropeptides.* 1988;11(1):17-21.

[44] Machado JD, Morales A, Gomez JF, Borges R. cAmp modulates exocytotic kinetics and increases quantal size in chromaffin cells. *Mol Pharmacol.* 2001;60(3):514-20.

[45] Marley PD, Thomson KA. Regulation of cyclic AMP metabolism in bovine adrenal medullary cells. *Biochem Pharmacol.* 1992;44(11):2105-10.

[46] Marley PD, Thomson KA, Jachno K, Johnston MJ. Histamine-induced increases in cyclic AMP levels in bovine adrenal medullary cells. *Br J Pharmacol.* 1991;104(4):839-46.

[47] Carabelli V, Hernandez-Guijo JM, Baldelli P, Carbone E. Direct autocrine inhibition and cAMP-dependent potentiation of single L-

type Ca^{2+} channels in bovine chromaffin cells. *J Physiol.* 2001;532(Pt 1):73-90.

[48] Carabelli V, Giancippoli A, Baldelli P, Carbone E, Artalejo AR. Distinct potentiation of L-type currents and secretion by cAMP in rat chromaffin cells. *Biophys J.* 2003;85(2):1326-37.

[49] Cesetti T, Hernandez-Guijo JM, Baldelli P, Carabelli V, Carbone E. Opposite action of beta1- and beta2-adrenergic receptors on Ca(V)1 L-channel current in rat adrenal chromaffin cells. *J Neurosci.* 2003;23(1):73-83.

[50] Neher E. Vesicle pools and Ca^{2+} microdomains: new tools for understanding their roles in neurotransmitter release. *Neuron.* 1998;20(3):389-99.

[51] Tang KS, Tse A, Tse FW. Differential regulation of multiple populations of granules in rat adrenal chromaffin cells by culture duration and cyclic AMP. *J Neurochem.* 2005;92(5):1126-39.

[52] Mancia G, Grassi G. The autonomic nervous system and hypertension. *Circulation research.* 114(11):1804-14.

[53] Fung MM, Viveros OH, O'Connor DT. Diseases of the adrenal medulla. *Acta physiologica* (Oxford, England). 2008;192(2):325-35.

[54] Miranda-Ferreira R, de Pascual R, de Diego AM, Caricati-Neto A, Gandia L, Jurkiewicz A, et al. Single-vesicle catecholamine release has greater quantal content and faster kinetics in chromaffin cells from hypertensive, as compared with normotensive, rats. *The Journal of pharmacology and experimental therapeutics.* 2008;324(2):685-93.

[55] Miranda-Ferreira R, de Pascual R, Caricati-Neto A, Gandia L, Jurkiewicz A, Garcia AG. Role of the endoplasmic reticulum and mitochondria on quantal catecholamine release from chromaffin cells of control and hypertensive rats. *The Journal of pharmacology and experimental therapeutics.* 2009;329(1):231-40.

[56] Miranda-Ferreira R, de Pascual R, Smaili SS, Caricati-Neto A, Gandia L, Garcia AG, et al. Greater cytosolic and mitochondrial calcium transients in adrenal medullary slices of hypertensive,

compared with normotensive rats. *European journal of pharmacology*. 636(1-3):126-36.

[57] Juszczak K, Drewa T. Adrenergic crisis due to pheochromocytoma - practical aspects. A short review. *Central European journal of urology*. 67(2):153-5.

[58] Fujita T. Concept of paraneurons. *Archivum histologicum Japonicum = Nihon soshikigaku kiroku.* 1977;40 Suppl:1-12.

[59] Livett BG. Adrenal medullary chromaffin cells *in vitro*. *Physiological reviews*. 1984;64(4):1103-61.

[60] Moro MA, Garcia AG, Langley OK. Characterization of two chromaffin cell populations isolated from bovine adrenal medulla. *Journal of neurochemistry*. 1991;57(2):363-9.

[61] Moro MA, Lopez MG, Gandia L, Michelena P, Garcia AG. Separation and culture of living adrenaline- and noradrenaline-containing cells from bovine adrenal medullae. *Analytical biochemistry*. 1990;185(2):243-8.

[62] Weiss JL. $Ca^{(2+)}$ signaling mechanisms in bovine adrenal chromaffin cells. *Advances in experimental medicine and biology.* 740:859-72.

[63] Douglas WW, Rubin RP. The role of calcium in the secretory response of the adrenal medulla to acetylcholine. *The Journal of physiology.* 1961;159:40-57.

[64] Burgoyne RD, Morgan A. Secretory granule exocytosis. *Physiological reviews*. 2003;83(2):581-632.

[65] Livett BG. Chromaffin cells: roles for vesicle proteins and Ca^{2+} in hormone secretion and exocytosis. *Trends in pharmacological sciences.* 1993;14(10):345-8.

[66] Cheek TR, Barry VA. Stimulus-secretion coupling in excitable cells: a central role for calcium. *The Journal of experimental biology*. 1993;184:183-96.

[67] Aunis D. Exocytosis in chromaffin cells of the adrenal medulla. *International review of cytology*. 1998;181:213-320.

[68] Penner R, Neher E. The role of calcium in stimulus-secretion coupling in excitable and non-excitable cells. *The Journal of experimental biology*. 1988;139:329-45.

[69] Garcia-Sancho J, Verkhratsky A. Cytoplasmic organelles determine complexity and specificity of calcium signalling in adrenal chromaffin cells. *Acta physiologica* (Oxford, England). 2008;192(2):263-71.

[70] Garcia-Sancho J. The coupling of plasma membrane calcium entry to calcium uptake by endoplasmic reticulum and mitochondria. *The Journal of physiology*. 592(Pt 2):261-8.

[71] Caricati-Neto A, Padin JF, Silva-Junior ED, Fernandez-Morales JC, de Diego AM, Jurkiewicz A, et al. Novel features on the regulation by mitochondria of calcium and secretion transients in chromaffin cells challenged with acetylcholine at 37 degrees C. *Physiol Rep.* 2013;1(7):e00182.

[72] Shimomura O. Preparation and handling of aequorin solutions for the measurement of cellular Ca^{2+}. *Cell calcium*. 1991;12(9):635-43.

[73] Shimomura O. The discovery of aequorin and green fluorescent protein. *Journal of microscopy*. 2005;217(Pt 1):1-15.

[74] Rizzuto R, Simpson AW, Brini M, Pozzan T. Rapid changes of mitochondrial Ca^{2+} revealed by specifically targeted recombinant aequorin. *Nature*. 1992;358(6384):325-7.

[75] Rizzuto R, Brini M, Pozzan T. Targeting recombinant aequorin to specific intracellular organelles. *Methods in cell biology*. 1994;40:339-58.

[76] Brini M, Pinton P, Pozzan T, Rizzuto R. Targeted recombinant aequorins: tools for monitoring (Ca^{2+}) in the various compartments of a living cell. *Microscopy research and technique*. 1999;46(6):380-9.

[77] Spaete RR, Frenkel N. The herpes simplex virus amplicon: a new eucaryotic defective-virus cloning-amplifying vector. *Cell.* 1982;30(1):295-304.

[78] Alonso MT, Barrero MJ, Carnicero E, Montero M, Garcia-Sancho J, Alvarez J. Functional measurements of (Ca^{2+}) in the endoplasmic reticulum using a herpes virus to deliver targeted aequorin. *Cell calcium*. 1998;24(2):87-96.

[79] Villalobos C, Nunez L, Chamero P, Alonso MT, Garcia-Sancho J. Mitochondrial ($Ca^{(2+)}$) oscillations driven by local high ($Ca^{(2+)}$)

domains generated by spontaneous electric activity. *The Journal of biological chemistry.* 2001;276(43):40293-7.

[80] Briggs CA, McAfee DA, McCaman RE. Long-term regulation of synaptic acetylcholine release and nicotinic transmission: the role of cyclic AMP. *British journal of pharmacology.* 1988;93(2):399-411.

[81] Kuba K, Kumamoto E. Long-term potentiation of transmitter release induced by adrenaline in bull-frog sympathetic ganglia. *The Journal of physiology.* 1986;374:515-30.

[82] Braas KM, Rossignol TM, Girard BM, May V, Parsons RL. Pituitary adenylate cyclase activating polypeptide (PACAP) decreases neuronal somatostatin immunoreactivity in cultured guinea-pig parasympathetic cardiac ganglia. *Neuroscience. 2004;126(2):335-46.*

[83] Chern YJ, Kim KT, Slakey LL, Westhead EW. Adenosine receptors activate adenylate cyclase and enhance secretion from bovine adrenal chromaffin cells in the presence of forskolin. *Journal of neurochemistry.* 1988;50(5):1484-93.

[84] Doyle ME, Egan JM. Pharmacological agents that directly modulate insulin secretion. *Pharmacological reviews.* 2003;55(1):105-31.

[85] Seino S, Shibasaki T. PKA-dependent and PKA-independent pathways for cAMP-regulated exocytosis. *Physiological reviews.* 2005;85(4):1303-42.

[86] Tang KS, Wang N, Tse A, Tse FW. Influence of quantal size and cAMP on the kinetics of quantal catecholamine release from rat chromaffin cells. *Biophysical journal.* 2007;92(8):2735-46.

[87] Bader MF, Holz RW, Kumakura K, Vitale N. Exocytosis: the chromaffin cell as a model system. *Annals of the New York Academy of Sciences.* 2002;971:178-83.

[88] Neher E. A comparison between exocytic control mechanisms in adrenal chromaffin cells and a glutamatergic synapse. *Pflugers Arch.* 2006;453(3):261-8.

[89] Burgoyne RD, Morgan A. Calcium sensors in regulated exocytosis. *Cell calcium.* 1998;24(5-6):367-76.

[90] Rigual R, Montero M, Rico AJ, Prieto-Lloret J, Alonso MT, Alvarez J. Modulation of secretion by the endoplasmic reticulum in mouse

chromaffin cells. *The European journal of neuroscience.* 2002;16(9):1690-6.

[91] Stevens DR, Schirra C, Becherer U, Rettig J. Vesicle pools: lessons from adrenal chromaffin cells. *Frontiers in synaptic neuroscience.* 3:2.

[92] Albillos A, Gil A, Gonzalez-Velez V, Perez-Alvarez A, Segura J, Hernandez-Vivanco A, et al. Exocytotic dynamics in human chromaffin cells: experiments and modeling. *Journal of computational neuroscience.* 34(1):27-37.

[93] Cuchillo-Ibanez I, Albillos A, Aldea M, Arroyo G, Fuentealba J, Garcia AG. Calcium entry, calcium redistribution, and exocytosis. *Annals of the New York Academy of Sciences.* 2002;971:108-16.

[94] Sasai M, Tadokoro S, Hirashima N. Artificial exocytotic system that secretes intravesicular contents upon Ca^{2+} influx. *Langmuir.* 26(18):14788-92.

[95] Izquierdo-Serra M, Trauner D, Llobet A, Gorostiza P. Optical control of calcium-regulated exocytosis. *Biochimica et biophysica acta.* 1830(3):2853-60.

[96] Zerbes M, Clark CL, Powis DA. Neurotransmitter release from bovine adrenal chromaffin cells is modulated by capacitative Ca(2+)entry driven by depleted internal $Ca^{(2+)}$stores. *Cell calcium.* 2001;29(1):49-58.

[97] Bartfai T, Iverfeldt K, Fisone G, Serfozo P. Regulation of the release of coexisting neurotransmitters. *Annual review of pharmacology and toxicology.* 1988;28:285-310.

[98] Lundberg JM. Peptide and classical transmitter mechanisms in the autonomic nervous system. *Archives internationales de pharmacodynamie et de therapie.* 1990;303:9-19. [*International Archives of Pharmacodynamics and Therapy.*]

[99] Golding DW. A pattern confirmed and refined--synaptic, nonsynaptic and parasynaptic exocytosis. *Bioessays.* 1994;16(7):503-8.

[100] Reetz A, Solimena M, Matteoli M, Folli F, Takei K, De Camilli P. GABA and pancreatic beta-cells: colocalization of glutamic acid decarboxylase (GAD) and GABA with synaptic-like microvesicles

suggests their role in GABA storage and secretion. *The EMBO journal.* 1991;10(5):1275-84.

[101] Michalik M, Erecinska M. GABA in pancreatic islets: metabolism and function. *Biochemical pharmacology.* 1992;44(1):1-9.

[102] MacDonald PE, Obermuller S, Vikman J, Galvanovskis J, Rorsman P, Eliasson L. Regulated exocytosis and kiss-and-run of synaptic-like microvesicles in INS-1 and primary rat beta-cells. *Diabetes.* 2005;54(3):736-43.

[103] Verhage M, McMahon HT, Ghijsen WE, Boomsma F, Scholten G, Wiegant VM, et al. Differential release of amino acids, neuropeptides, and catecholamines from isolated nerve terminals. *Neuron.* 1991;6(4):517-24.

[104] Sorenson RL, Garry DG, Brelje TC. Structural and functional considerations of GABA in islets of Langerhans. Beta-cells and nerves. *Diabetes.* 1991;40(11):1365-74.

[105] Satin LS, Kinard TA. Neurotransmitters and their receptors in the islets of Langerhans of the pancreas: what messages do acetylcholine, glutamate, and GABA transmit? *Endocrine.* 1998;8(3):213-23.

[106] Zhu PC, Thureson-Klein A, Klein RL. Exocytosis from large dense cored vesicles outside the active synaptic zones of terminals within the trigeminal subnucleus caudalis: a possible mechanism for neuropeptide release. *Neuroscience.* 1986;19(1):43-54.

[107] Wendt A, Birnir B, Buschard K, Gromada J, Salehi A, Sewing S, et al. Glucose inhibition of glucagon secretion from rat alpha-cells is mediated by GABA released from neighboring beta-cells. *Diabetes.* 2004;53(4):1038-45.

[108] Sudhof TC. The synaptic vesicle cycle. *Annual review of neuroscience.* 2004;27:509-47.

[109] Hille B, Billiard J, Babcock DF, Nguyen T, Koh DS. Stimulation of exocytosis without a calcium signal. *The Journal of physiology.* 1999;520 Pt 1:23-31.

[110] Aunis D, Langley K. Physiological aspects of exocytosis in chromaffin cells of the adrenal medulla. *Acta physiologica Scandinavica.* 1999;167(2):89-97.

[111] Borges R, Machado JD, Betancor G, Camacho M. Pharmacological regulation of the late steps of exocytosis. *Annals of the New York Academy of Sciences.* 2002;971:184-92.

[112] Burgess TL, Kelly RB. Constitutive and regulated secretion of proteins. *Annual review of cell biology.* 1987;3:243-93.

[113] Rettig J, Neher E. Emerging roles of presynaptic proteins in C^{a++}-triggered exocytosis. *Science* (New York, NY. 2002;298(5594): 781-5.

[114] Prentki M, Matschinsky FM. Ca^{2+}, cAMP, and phospholipid-derived messengers in coupling mechanisms of insulin secretion. *Physiological reviews.* 1987;67(4):1185-248.

[115] Byrne JH, Kandel ER. Presynaptic facilitation revisited: state and time dependence. *J Neurosci.* 1996;16(2):425-35.

[116] Kits KS, Mansvelder HD. Regulation of exocytosis in neuroendocrine cells: spatial organization of channels and vesicles, stimulus-secretion coupling, calcium buffers and modulation. *Brain research.* 2000;33(1):78-94.

[117] Calakos N, Scheller RH. Synaptic vesicle biogenesis, docking, and fusion: a molecular description. *Physiological reviews.* 1996;76(1):1-29.

[118] Augustine GJ, Burns ME, DeBello WM, Pettit DL, Schweizer FE. Exocytosis: proteins and perturbations. *Annual review of pharmacology and toxicology.* 1996;36:659-701.

[119] Baker PF, Knight DE. Calcium-dependent exocytosis in bovine adrenal medullary cells with leaky plasma membranes. *Nature.* 1978;276(5688):620-2.

[120] Holz RW, Bittner MA, Peppers SC, Senter RA, Eberhard DA. MgATP-independent and MgATP-dependent exocytosis. Evidence that MgATP primes adrenal chromaffin cells to undergo exocytosis. *The Journal of biological chemistry.* 1989;264(10):5412-9.

[121] Neher E, Zucker RS. Multiple calcium-dependent processes related to secretion in bovine chromaffin cells. *Neuron.* 1993;10(1):21-30.

[122] Carafoli E. The calcium cycle of mitochondria. *FEBS letters.* 1979;104(1):1-5.

[123] Duchen MR. Mitochondria and Ca($^{2+}$)in cell physiology and pathophysiology. *Cell calcium.* 2000;28(5-6):339-48.

[124] Duchen MR, Szabadkai G. Roles of mitochondria in human disease. *Essays in biochemistry.* 47:115-37.

[125] Villalobos C, Nunez L, Montero M, Garcia AG, Alonso MT, Chamero P, et al. Redistribution of Ca^{2+} among cytosol and organella during stimulation of bovine chromaffin cells. *Faseb J.* 2002;16(3):343-53.

[126] Rizzuto R, Brini M, Murgia M, Pozzan T. Microdomains with high Ca^{2+} close to IP3-sensitive channels that are sensed by neighboring mitochondria. *Science* (New York, NY. 1993;262(5134):744-7.

[127] Babcock DF, Herrington J, Goodwin PC, Park YB, Hille B. Mitochondrial participation in the intracellular Ca^{2+} network. *The Journal of cell biology.* 1997;136(4):833-44.

[128] Xu T, Naraghi M, Kang H, Neher E. Kinetic studies of Ca^{2+} binding and Ca^{2+} clearance in the cytosol of adrenal chromaffin cells. *Biophysical journal.* 1997;73(1):532-45.

[129] Montero M, Alonso MT, Carnicero E, Cuchillo-Ibanez I, Albillos A, Garcia AG, et al. Chromaffin-cell stimulation triggers fast millimolar mitochondrial Ca^{2+} transients that modulate secretion. *Nature cell biology.* 2000;2(2):57-61.

[130] Kao LS, Cheung NS. Mechanism of calcium transport across the plasma membrane of bovine chromaffin cells. *Journal of neurochemistry.* 1990;54(6):1972-9.

[131] Salvador JM, Inesi G, Rigaud JL, Mata AM. Ca^{2+} transport by reconstituted synaptosomal ATPase is associated with H+ countertransport and net charge displacement. *The Journal of biological chemistry.* 1998;273(29):18230-4.

[132] Baker PF, Blaustein MP, Hodgkin AL, Steinhardt RA. The influence of calcium on sodium efflux in squid axons. *The Journal of physiology.* 1969;200(2):431-58.

[133] Blaustein MP, Lederer WJ. Sodium/calcium exchange: its physiological implications. *Physiological reviews.* 1999;79(3):763-854.

[134] Annunziato L, Pignataro G, Di Renzo GF. Pharmacology of brain Na^+/Ca^{2+} exchanger: from molecular biology to therapeutic perspectives. *Pharmacological reviews.* 2004;56(4):633-54.

[135] Pan CY, Kao LS. Catecholamine secretion from bovine adrenal chromaffin cells: the role of the $Na+/Ca^{2+}$ exchanger and the intracellular Ca^{2+} pool. *Journal of neurochemistry.* 1997;69(3):1085-92.

[136] Pan CY, Chu YS, Kao LS. Molecular study of the $Na+/Ca^{2+}$ exchanger in bovine adrenal chromaffin cells. *The Biochemical journal.* 1998;336 (Pt 2):305-10.

[137] Liu PS, Kao LS. Na(+)-dependent Ca^{2+} influx in bovine adrenal chromaffin cells. *Cell calcium.* 1990;11(9):573-9.

[138] Powis DA, O'Brien KJ, Von Grafenstein HR. Calcium export by sodium-calcium exchange in bovine chromaffin cells. *Cell calcium.* 1991;12(7):493-504.

[139] Pan CY, Huang CH, Lee CH. Calcium elevation elicited by reverse mode Na^+/Ca^{2+} exchange activity is facilitated by intracellular calcium stores in bovine chromaffin cells. *Biochemical and biophysical research communications.* 2006;342(2):589-95.

[140] Berridge MJ. Calcium microdomains: organization and function. *Cell calcium.* 2006;40(5-6):405-12.

[141] Harr MW, Distelhorst CW. Apoptosis and autophagy: decoding calcium signals that mediate life or death. *Cold Spring Harbor perspectives in biology.* 2(10):a005579.

[142] De Crescenzo V, ZhuGe R, Velazquez-Marrero C, Lifshitz LM, Custer E, Carmichael J, et al. Ca^{2+} syntillas, miniature Ca^{2+} release events in terminals of hypothalamic neurons, are increased in frequency by depolarization in the absence of Ca^{2+} influx. *J Neurosci.* 2004;24(5):1226-35.

[143] ZhuGe R, DeCrescenzo V, Sorrentino V, Lai FA, Tuft RA, Lifshitz LM, et al. Syntillas release Ca^{2+} at a site different from the microdomain where exocytosis occurs in mouse chromaffin cells. *Biophysical journal.* 2006;90(6):2027-37.

[144] Lefkowitz JJ, Fogarty KE, Lifshitz LM, Bellve KD, Tuft RA, ZhuGe R, et al. Suppression of Ca^{2+} syntillas increases spontaneous exocytosis in mouse adrenal chromaffin cells. *The Journal of general physiology.* 2009;134(4):267-80.

[145] Alonso MT, Barrero MJ, Michelena P, Carnicero E, Cuchillo I, Garcia AG, et al. Ca^{2+}-induced Ca^{2+} release in chromaffin cells seen from inside the ER with targeted aequorin. *The Journal of cell biology.* 1999;144(2):241-54.

[146] Zhou Z, Neher E. Mobile and immobile calcium buffers in bovine adrenal chromaffin cells. *The Journal of physiology.* 1993;469:245-73.

[147] Artalejo CR, Garcia AG, Aunis D. Chromaffin cell calcium channel kinetics measured isotopically through fast calcium, strontium, and barium fluxes. *The Journal of biological chemistry.* 1987;262(2):915-26.

[148] Naraghi M, Muller TH, Neher E. Two-dimensional determination of the cellular Ca^{2+} binding in bovine chromaffin cells. *Biophysical journal.* 1998;75(4):1635-47.

[149] Neher E, Augustine GJ. Calcium gradients and buffers in bovine chromaffin cells. *The Journal of physiology.* 1992;450:273-301.

[150] Neher E. Usefulness and limitations of linear approximations to the understanding of Ca^{++} signals. *Cell calcium.* 1998;24(5-6):345-57.

[151] Hernandez-Cruz A, Sala F, Adams PR. Subcellular calcium transients visualized by confocal microscopy in a voltage-clamped vertebrate neuron. *Science* (New York, NY. 1990;247(4944):858-62.

[152] Alonso MT, Chamero P, Villalobos C, Garcia-Sancho J. Fura-2 antagonises calcium-induced calcium release. *Cell calcium.* 2003;33(1):27-35.

[153] Nowycky MC, Pinter MJ. Time courses of calcium and calcium-bound buffers following calcium influx in a model cell. *Biophysical journal.* 1993;64(1):77-91.

[154] Herrington J, Park YB, Babcock DF, Hille B. Dominant role of mitochondria in clearance of large Ca^{2+} loads from rat adrenal chromaffin cells. *Neuron.* 1996;16(1):219-28.

[155] Gunter TE, Pfeiffer DR. Mechanisms by which mitochondria transport calcium. *The American journal of physiology*. 1990;258(5 Pt 1):C755-86.

[156] Montero M, Alonso MT, Albillos A, Garcia-Sancho J, Alvarez J. Mitochondrial Ca^{2+}-induced Ca^{2+} release mediated by the Ca^{2+} uniporter. *Molecular biology of the cell*. 2001;12(1):63-71.

[157] Uceda G, Garcia AG, Guantes JM, Michelena P, Montiel C. Effects of Ca^{2+} channel antagonist subtypes on mitochondrial Ca^{2+} transport. *European journal of pharmacology*. 1995;289(1):73-80.

[158] Park YB, Herrington J, Babcock DF, Hille B. Ca^{2+} clearance mechanisms in isolated rat adrenal chromaffin cells. *The Journal of physiology*. 1996;492 (Pt 2):329-46.

[159] von Ruden L, Neher E. A Ca-dependent early step in the release of catecholamines from adrenal chromaffin cells. *Science* (New York, NY. 1993;262(5136):1061-5.

[160] Chow RH, Klingauf J, Neher E. Time course of Ca^{2+} concentration triggering exocytosis in neuroendocrine cells. *Proceedings of the National Academy of Sciences of the United States of America*. 1994;91(26):12765-9.

[161] Klingauf J, Neher E. Modeling buffered Ca^{2+} diffusion near the membrane: implications for secretion in neuroendocrine cells. *Biophysical journal*. 1997;72(2 Pt 1):674-90.

[162] Robinson IM, Yamada M, Carrion-Vazquez M, Lennon VA, Fernandez JM. Specialized release zones in chromaffin cells examined with pulsed-laser imaging. *Cell calcium*. 1996;20(2):181-201.

[163] Zhou Z, Misler S. Action potential-induced quantal secretion of catecholamines from rat adrenal chromaffin cells. *The Journal of biological chemistry*. 1995;270(8):3498-505.

[164] Olivos Ore L, Artalejo AR. Intracellular Ca^{2+} microdomain-triggered exocytosis in neuroendocrine cells. *Trends in neurosciences*. 2004;27(3):113-5.

[165] Becherer U, Moser T, Stuhmer W, Oheim M. Calcium regulates exocytosis at the level of single vesicles. *Nature neuroscience.* 2003;6(8):846-53.

[166] Westerink RH. Exocytosis: using amperometry to study presynaptic mechanisms of neurotoxicity. *Neurotoxicology.* 2004;25(3):461-70.

[167] Bittner MA, Holz RW. Kinetic analysis of secretion from permeabilized adrenal chromaffin cells reveals distinct components. *The Journal of biological chemistry.* 1992;267(23):16219-25.

[168] Heinemann C, von Ruden L, Chow RH, Neher E. A two-step model of secretion control in neuroendocrine cells. *Pflugers Arch.* 1993;424(2):105-12.

[169] Cochilla AJ, Angleson JK, Betz WJ. Differential regulation of granule-to-granule and granule-to-plasma membrane fusion during secretion from rat pituitary lactotrophs. *The Journal of cell biology.* 2000;150(4):839-48.

[170] Fujita-Yoshigaki J. Divergence and convergence in regulated exocytosis: the characteristics of cAMP-dependent enzyme secretion of parotid salivary acinar cells. *Cellular signalling.* 1998;10(6): 371-5.

[171] Kuromi H, Kidokoro Y. Two synaptic vesicle pools, vesicle recruitment and replenishment of pools at the Drosophila neuromuscular junction. *Journal of neurocytology.* 2003;32(5-8):551-65.

[172] Leech CA, Holz GG, Habener JF. Signal transduction of PACAP and GLP-1 in pancreatic beta cells. *Annals of the New York Academy of Sciences.* 1996;805:81-92; discussion -3.

[173] Lonart G, Janz R, Johnson KM, Sudhof TC. Mechanism of action of rab3A in mossy fiber LTP. *Neuron.* 1998;21(5):1141-50.

[174] Malaisse WJ, Malaisse-Lagae F. The role of cyclic AMP in insulin release. *Experientia.* 1984;40(10):1068-74.

[175] Muto Y, Nagao T, Yamada M, Mikoshiba K, Urushidani T. A proposed mechanism for the potentiation of cAMP-mediated acid secretion by carbachol. *American journal of physiology.* 2001;280(1):C155-65.

[176] Sakaba T, Neher E. Preferential potentiation of fast-releasing synaptic vesicles by cAMP at the calyx of Held. *Proceedings of the National Academy of Sciences of the United States of America.* 2001;98(1):331-6.

[177] Sato K, Ohsaga A, Oshiro T, Ito S, Maruyama Y. Involvement of GTP-binding protein in pancreatic cAMP-mediated exocytosis. *Pflugers Arch.* 2002;443(3):394-8.

[178] Trudeau LE, Fang Y, Haydon PG. Modulation of an early step in the secretory machinery in hippocampal nerve terminals. *Proceedings of the National Academy of Sciences of the United States of America.* 1998;95(12):7163-8.

[179] Bliss TV, Collingridge GL. A synaptic model of memory: long-term potentiation in the hippocampus. *Nature.* 1993;361(6407):31-9.

[180] Larkman AU, Jack JJ. Synaptic plasticity: hippocampal LTP. *Current opinion in neurobiology.* 1995;5(3):324-34.

[181] Nicoll RA, Malenka RC. Contrasting properties of two forms of long-term potentiation in the hippocampus. *Nature.* 1995;377(6545):115-8.

[182] Trudeau LE, Emery DG, Haydon PG. Direct modulation of the secretory machinery underlies PKA-dependent synaptic facilitation in hippocampal neurons. *Neuron.* 1996;17(4):789-97.

[183] Weisskopf MG, Castillo PE, Zalutsky RA, Nicoll RA. Mediation of hippocampal mossy fiber long-term potentiation by cyclic AMP. *Science* (New York, NY. 1994;265(5180):1878-82.

[184] Chen C, Regehr WG. The mechanism of cAMP-mediated enhancement at a cerebellar synapse. *J Neurosci.* 1997;17(22):8687-94.

[185] Salin PA, Malenka RC, Nicoll RA. Cyclic AMP mediates a presynaptic form of LTP at cerebellar parallel fiber synapses. *Neuron.* 1996;16(4):797-803.

[186] Silveira WA, Goncalves DA, Graca FA, Andrade-Lopes AL, Bergantin LB, Zanon NM, et al. Activating cAMP/PKA signaling in skeletal muscle suppresses the ubiquitin-proteasome-dependent

proteolysis: implications for sympathetic regulation. *J Appl Physiol* (1985). 2014;117(1):11-9.

[187] Zhong N, Zucker RS. Roles of Ca^{2+}, hyperpolarization and cyclic nucleotide-activated channel activation, and actin in temporal synaptic tagging. *J Neurosci.* 2004;24(17):4205-12.

[188] Brunelli M, Castellucci V, Kandel ER. Synaptic facilitation and behavioral sensitization in Aplysia: possible role of serotonin and cyclic AMP. *Science* (New York, NY. 1976;194(4270):1178-81.

[189] Castellucci VF, Kandel ER, Schwartz JH, Wilson FD, Nairn AC, Greengard P. Intracellular injection of the catalytic subunit of cyclic AMP-dependent protein kinase simulates facilitation of transmitter release underlying behavioral sensitization in Aplysia. *Proceedings of the National Academy of Sciences of the United States of America.* 1980;77(12):7492-6.

[190] Kandel ER, Schwartz JH. Molecular biology of learning: modulation of transmitter release. *Science* (New York, NY. 1982;218 (4571):433-43.

[191] Klein M. Differential cyclic AMP dependence of facilitation at Aplysia sensorimotor synapses as a function of prior stimulation: augmentation versus restoration of transmitter release. *J Neurosci.* 1993;13(9):3793-801.

[192] Shuster MJ, Camardo JS, Siegelbaum SA, Kandel ER. Cyclic AMP-dependent protein kinase closes the serotonin-sensitive K^+ channels of Aplysia sensory neurones in cell-free membrane patches. *Nature.* 1985;313(6001):392-5.

[193] Yoshihara M, Suzuki K, Kidokoro Y. Two independent pathways mediated by cAMP and protein kinase A enhance spontaneous transmitter release at Drosophila neuromuscular junctions. *J Neurosci.* 2000;20(22):8315-22.

[194] Bratanova-Tochkova TK, Cheng H, Daniel S, Gunawardana S, Liu YJ, Mulvaney-Musa J, et al. Triggering and augmentation mechanisms, granule pools, and biphasic insulin secretion. *Diabetes.* 2002;51 Suppl 1:S83-90.

[195] Hedeskov CJ. Mechanism of glucose-induced insulin secretion. *Physiological reviews*. 1980;60(2):442-509.
[196] Henquin JC. The interplay between cyclic AMP and ions in the stimulus-secretion coupling in pancreatic B-cells. *Archives internationales de physiologie et de biochimie*. 1985;93(1):37-48. [*International Archives of Physiology and Biochemistry*]
[197] Sharp GW. The adenylate cyclase-cyclic AMP system in islets of Langerhans and its role in the control of insulin release. *Diabetologia*. 1979;16(5):287-96.
[198] Sutherland EW, Robison GA. The role of cyclic AMP in the control of carbohydrate metabolism. *Diabetes*. 1969;18(12):797-819.
[199] Ding WG, Renstrom E, Rorsman P, Buschard K, Gromada J. Glucagon-like peptide I and glucose-dependent insulinotropic polypeptide stimulate Ca^{2+}-induced secretion in rat alpha-cells by a protein kinase A-mediated mechanism. *Diabetes*. 1997;46(5):792-800.
[200] Gromada J, Bokvist K, Ding WG, Barg S, Buschard K, Renstrom E, et al. Adrenaline stimulates glucagon secretion in pancreatic A-cells by increasing the Ca^{2+} current and the number of granules close to the L-type Ca^{2+} channels. *The Journal of general physiology*. 1997;110(3):217-28.
[201] Antoni FA, Sosunov AA, Haunso A, Paterson JM, Simpson J. Short-term plasticity of cyclic adenosine 3',5'-monophosphate signaling in anterior pituitary corticotrope cells: the role of adenylyl cyclase isotypes. *Molecular endocrinology* (Baltimore, Md. 2003;17(4):692-703.
[202] Luini A, Lewis D, Guild S, Corda D, Axelrod J. Hormone secretagogues increase cytosolic calcium by increasing cAMP in corticotropin-secreting cells. *Proceedings of the National Academy of Sciences of the United States of America*. 1985;82(23):8034-8.
[203] Won JG, Orth DN. Roles of intracellular and extracellular calcium in the kinetic profile of adrenocorticotropin secretion by perifused rat anterior pituitary cells. I. Corticotropin-releasing factor stimulation. *Endocrinology*. 1990;126(2):849-57.

[204] Silveira WA, Goncalves DA, Graca FA, Andrade-Lopes AL, Bergantin LB, Zanon NM, et al. Activating cAMP/PKA signaling in skeletal muscle suppresses the ubiquitin-proteasome-dependent proteolysis: implications for sympathetic regulation. *J Appl Physiol* (1985).117(1):11-9.

[205] Bergantin LB, Andrade-Lopes AL, Chiavegatti T, Godinho RO. Effects of Chronic Denervation on Adenylyl Cyclase Activity of Fast and Slow Twitch Muscles. *Journal of Molecular Neuroscience.* 2010;40(1-2):236-7.

[206] Quissell DO, Barzen KA, Deisher LM. Rat submandibular and parotid protein phosphorylation and exocytosis: effect of site-selective cAMP analogs. *Crit Rev Oral Biol Med*. 1993;4(3-4):443-8.

[207] Kaupp UB, Seifert R. Cyclic nucleotide-gated ion channels. *Physiological reviews*. 2002;82(3):769-824.

[208] Biel M, Schneider A, Wahl C. Cardiac HCN channels: structure, function, and modulation. *Trends in cardiovascular medicine.* 2002;12(5):206-12.

[209] Bos JL. Epac: a new cAMP target and new avenues in cAMP research. *Nature reviews*. 2003;4(9):733-8.

[210] Springett GM, Kawasaki H, Spriggs DR. Non-kinase second-messenger signaling: new pathways with new promise. *Bioessays.* 2004;26(7):730-8.

[211] Cooper DM, Mons N, Karpen JW. Adenylyl cyclases and the interaction between calcium and cAMP signalling. *Nature.* 1995;374(6521):421-4.

[212] Halls ML, Cooper DM. Regulation by Ca^{2+}-signaling pathways of adenylyl cyclases. *Cold Spring Harb Perspect Biol.* 2011;3(1):a004143.

[213] Antoni FA. Interactions between intracellular free Ca^{2+} and cyclic AMP in neuroendocrine cells. *Cell calcium*. 51(3-4):260-6.

[214] Willoughby D. Organization of cAMP signalling microdomains for optimal regulation by Ca^{2+} entry. *Biochem Soc Trans.* 2012;40(1):246-50.

[215] Fagan KA, Graf RA, Tolman S, Schaack J, Cooper DM. Regulation of a Ca2+-sensitive adenylyl cyclase in an excitable cell. Role of voltage-gated versus capacitative Ca^{2+} entry. *J Biol Chem.* 2000;275(51):40187-94.

[216] Bender AT, Beavo JA. Cyclic nucleotide phosphodiesterases: molecular regulation to clinical use. *Pharmacol Rev.* 2006;58(3):488-520.

[217] Goraya TA, Masada N, Ciruela A, Willoughby D, Clynes MA, Cooper DM. Kinetic properties of Ca^{2+}/calmodulin-dependent phosphodiesterase isoforms dictate intracellular cAMP dynamics in response to elevation of cytosolic Ca^{2+}. *Cell Signal.* 2008;20(2):359-74.

[218] Giovannucci DR, Groblewski GE, Sneyd J, Yule DI. Targeted phosphorylation of inositol 1,4,5-trisphosphate receptors selectively inhibits localized Ca^{2+} release and shapes oscillatory Ca^{2+} signals. *J Biol Chem.* 2000;275(43):33704-11.

[219] Marks AR. Calcium cycling proteins and heart failure: mechanisms and therapeutics. *J Clin Invest.* 2013;123(1):46-52.

[220] Fuller MD, Emrick MA, Sadilek M, Scheuer T, Catterall WA. Molecular mechanism of calcium channel regulation in the fight-or-flight response. *Sci Signal.* 2010;3(141):ra70.

[221] Wang H, Zhang M. The role of Ca(2)(+)-stimulated adenylyl cyclases in bidirectional synaptic plasticity and brain function. *Rev Neurosci.* 2012;23(1):67-78.

[222] Wagner LE, 2nd, Joseph SK, Yule DI. Regulation of single inositol 1,4,5-trisphosphate receptor channel activity by protein kinase A phosphorylation. *J Physiol.* 2008;586(Pt 15):3577-96.

[223] Lanner JT, Georgiou DK, Joshi AD, Hamilton SL. Ryanodine receptors: structure, expression, molecular details, and function in calcium release. *Cold Spring Harb Perspect Biol.* 2010;2(11):a003996.

[224] Yule DI, Betzenhauser MJ, Joseph SK. Linking structure to function: Recent lessons from inositol 1,4,5-trisphosphate receptor mutagenesis. *Cell Calcium.* 2010;47(6):469-79.

[225] Bittner MA, Holz RW. Phorbol esters enhance exocytosis from chromaffin cells by two mechanisms. *Journal of neurochemistry.* 1990;54(1):205-10.

[226] Brocklehurst KW, Pollard HB. Enhancement of Ca^{2+}-induced catecholamine release by the phorbol ester TPA in digitonin-permeabilized cultured bovine adrenal chromaffin cells. *FEBS letters. 1985;183(1):107-10.*

[227] Burgoyne RD, Morgan A, O'Sullivan AJ. A major role for protein kinase C in calcium-activated exocytosis in permeabilised adrenal chromaffin cells. *FEBS letters.* 1988;238(1):151-5.

[228] Burgoyne RD, Norman KM. Effect of calmidazolium and phorbol ester on catecholamine secretion from adrenal chromaffin cells. *Biochimica et biophysica acta.* 1984;805(1):37-43. [*Biochemistry and Biophysics Journal*]

[229] Cuchillo-Ibanez I, Lejen T, Albillos A, Rose SD, Olivares R, Villarroya M, et al. Mitochondrial calcium sequestration and protein kinase C cooperate in the regulation of cortical F-actin disassembly and secretion in bovine chromaffin cells. *The Journal of physiology.* 2004;560(Pt 1):63-76.

[230] Burgoyne RD, Morgan A, O'Sullivan AJ. The control of cytoskeletal actin and exocytosis in intact and permeabilized adrenal chromaffin cells: role of calcium and protein kinase C. *Cellular signalling.* 1989;1(4):323-34.

[231] Cheek TR, Burgoyne RD. Cyclic AMP inhibits both nicotine-induced actin disassembly and catecholamine secretion from bovine adrenal chromaffin cells. *The Journal of biological chemistry.* 1987;262(24):11663-6.

[232] Cheek TR, Burgoyne RD. Nicotine-evoked disassembly of cortical actin filaments in adrenal chromaffin cells. *FEBS letters.* 1986;207(1):110-4.

[233] Vitale ML, Seward EP, Trifaro JM. Chromaffin cell cortical actin network dynamics control the size of the release-ready vesicle pool and the initial rate of exocytosis. *Neuron.* 1995;14(2):353-63.

[234] Vitale ML, Rodriguez Del Castillo A, Trifaro JM. Protein kinase C activation by phorbol esters induces chromaffin cell cortical filamentous actin disassembly and increases the initial rate of exocytosis in response to nicotinic receptor stimulation. *Neuroscience.* 1992;51(2):463-74.

[235] Gillis KD, Mossner R, Neher E. Protein kinase C enhances exocytosis from chromaffin cells by increasing the size of the readily releasable pool of secretory granules. *Neuron.* 1996;16(6):1209-20.

[236] Smith C, Moser T, Xu T, Neher E. Cytosolic Ca^{2+} acts by two separate pathways to modulate the supply of release-competent vesicles in chromaffin cells. *Neuron.* 1998;20(6):1243-53.

[237] Smith C. A persistent activity-dependent facilitation in chromaffin cells is caused by Ca^{2+} activation of protein kinase C. *J Neurosci.* 1999;19(2):589-98.

[238] Duncan RR, Betz A, Shipston MJ, Brose N, Chow RH. Transient, phorbol ester-induced DOC2-Munc13 interactions *in vivo*. *The Journal of biological chemistry.* 1999;274(39):27347-50.

[239] Barclay JW, Craig TJ, Fisher RJ, Ciufo LF, Evans GJ, Morgan A, et al. Phosphorylation of Munc18 by protein kinase C regulates the kinetics of exocytosis. *The Journal of biological chemistry.* 2003;278(12):10538-45.

[240] Nagy G, Matti U, Nehring RB, Binz T, Rettig J, Neher E, et al. Protein kinase C-dependent phosphorylation of synaptosome-associated protein of 25 kDa at Ser187 potentiates vesicle recruitment. *J Neurosci.* 2002;22(21):9278-86.

[241] Sudhof TC. The synaptic vesicle cycle: a cascade of protein-protein interactions. *Nature.* 1995;375(6533):645-53.

[242] Ohara-Imaizumi M, Fukuda M, Niinobe M, Misonou H, Ikeda K, Murakami T, et al. Distinct roles of C2A and C2B domains of synaptotagmin in the regulation of exocytosis in adrenal chromaffin cells. *Proceedings of the National Academy of Sciences of the United States of America.* 1997;94(1):287-91.

[243] Trifaro JM, Fournier S, Novas ML. The p65 protein is a calmodulin-binding protein present in several types of secretory vesicles. *Neuroscience.* 1989;29(1):1-8.

[244] Elhamdani A, Martin TF, Kowalchyk JA, Artalejo CR. Ca$^{(2+)}$-dependent activator protein for secretion is critical for the fusion of dense-core vesicles with the membrane in calf adrenal chromaffin cells. *J Neurosci.* 1999;19(17):7375-83.

[245] Zamponi GW. Targeting voltage-gated calcium channels in neurological and psychiatric diseases. *Nat Rev Drug Discov.* 2016;15(1):19-34.

[246] Kaster MP, Moretti M, Cunha MP, Rodrigues AL. Novel approaches for the management of depressive disorders. *Eur J Pharmacol.* 2016;771:236-40.

[247] Salat D, Noyce AJ, Schrag A, Tolosa E. Challenges of modifying disease progression in prediagnostic Parkinson's disease. *Lancet Neurol.* 2016.

[248] Mohamed T, Shakeri A, Rao PP. Amyloid cascade in Alzheimer's disease: Recent advances in medicinal chemistry. *Eur J Med Chem.* 2016;113:258-72.

[249] Maroto M, de Diego AM, Albinana E, Fernandez-Morales JC, Caricati-Neto A, Jurkiewicz A, et al. Multi-target novel neuroprotective compound ITH33/IQM9.21 inhibits calcium entry, calcium signals and exocytosis. *Cell Calcium.* 2011;50(4):359-69.

[250] Kawamoto EM, Vivar C, Camandola S. Physiology and pathology of calcium signaling in the brain. *Front Pharmacol.* 2012;3:61.

[251] Ismaili L, Refouvelet B, Benchekroun M, Brogi S, Brindisi M, Gemma S, et al. Multitarget compounds bearing tacrine- and donepezil-like structural and functional motifs for the potential treatment of Alzheimer's disease. *Prog Neurobiol.* 2016.

[252] Mathis S, Couratier P, Julian A, Vallat JM, Corcia P, Le Masson G (2016). Management and therapeutic perspectives in amyotrophic lateral sclerosis. *Exp Rev Neurother.* 1–14.

[253] Rowland LP, Shneider NA (2001). Amyotrophic lateral sclerosis. *N Engl J Med.* 344:1688–1700.

[254] Chiò A, Logroscino G, Traynor BJ, et al. (2013). Global epidemiology of amyotrophic lateral sclerosis: a systematic review of the published literature. *Neuroepidemiology.* 41(2):118–30.
[255] Wang MD, Little J, Gomes J, et al. (2016). Identification of risk factors associated with onset and progression of amyotrophic lateral sclerosis using systematic review and meta-analysis. *Neurotoxicology*, pii: S0161-813X(16)30116-4.
[256] Sutedja NA, Veldink JH, Fischer K, et al. (2009). Exposure to chemicals and metals and risk of amyotrophic lateral sclerosis: a systematic review. *Amyotroph Lateral Scler.* 10(5–6):302–9.
[257] Delzor A, Couratier P, Boumédiène F, et al. (2014). Searching for a link between the L-BMAA neurotoxin and amyotrophic lateral sclerosis: a study protocol of the French BMAALS programme. *BMJ Open*, 4(8):e005528.
[258] Malek AM, Barchowsky A, Bowser R, et al. (2015). Exposure to hazardous air pollutants and the risk of amyotrophic lateral sclerosis. *Environ Pollut.,* 197:181–6.
[259] Bozzoni V, Pansarasa O, Diamanti L, et al. (2016). Amyotrophic lateral sclerosis and environmental factors. *Funct Neurol.,* 31(1):7–19.
[260] Rooney J, Vajda A, Heverin M, et al. (2016). No association between soil constituents and amyotrophic lateral sclerosis relative risk in Ireland. *Environ Res.* 147:102–7.
[261] Ilijic E, Guzman JN, Surmeier DJ (2011). The L-type channel antagonist isradipine is neuroprotective in a mouse model of Parkinson's disease. *Neurobiol Dis* 43(2): 364-71.
[262] Wu CL, Wen SH (2016). A 10-year follow-up study of the association between calcium channel blocker use and the risk of dementia in elderly hypertensive patients. *Medicine* (Baltimore) 95(32): e4593.
[263] Doble A (1996). The pharmacology and mechanism of action of riluzole. *Neurology,* 47:S233–241.
[264] Bergantin LB, Caricati-Neto A (2016) Challenges for the pharmacological treatment of neurological and psychiatric disorders:

Implications of the Ca^{2+}/cAMP intracellular signalling interaction. *Eur J Pharmacol* 788: 255-260.

[265] Bergantin LB, Caricati-Neto A (2016) Insight from "Calcium Paradox" due to Ca^{2+}/cAMP Interaction: Novel Pharmacological Strategies for the Treatment of Depression. *Int Arch Clin Pharmacol* 2: 007.

[266] Bergantin LB, Caricati-Neto A (2016) Novel Insights for Therapy of Parkinson's disease: Pharmacological Modulation of the Ca^{2+}/cAMP Signalling Interaction. *Austin Neurol & Neurosci* 1 (2): 1009.

[267] Bergantin LB, Caricati-Neto A (2016) Recent advances in pharmacotherapy of neurological and psychiatric disorders promoted by discovery of the role of Ca^{2+}/cAMP signaling interaction in the neurotransmission and neuroprotection. *Adv Pharmac J* 1(3): 66.

[268] Bergantin LB, Caricati-Neto A (2016) From discovering "calcium paradox" to Ca^{2+}/cAMP interaction: Impact in human health and disease. *Scholars Press* 120p.

[269] Bergantin LB, Caricati-Neto A (2016) New therapeutic strategy of Alzheimer's and Parkinson's diseases: Pharmacological modulation of neural Ca^{2+}/cAMP intracellular signaling interaction. *Asian Journal of Pharmacy and Pharmacology* 2(6): 136-143.

[270] Bergantin LB, Caricati-Neto A (2016) Impact of interaction of Ca^{2+}/cAMP Intracellular Signalling Pathways in Clinical Pharmacology and Translational Medicine. *Clinical Pharmacology and Translational Medicine*, 1-4.

[271] Bergantin LB, Caricati-Neto A (2016) Challenges for the Pharmacological Treatment of Dementia: Implications of the Ca^{2+}/cAMP Intracellular Signalling Interaction. *Avidscience*, 2-25.

[272] Bergantin, LB; Caricati-Neto A. The discovery of the 'calcium paradox' due to Ca^{2+}/cAMP interaction: novel adventures for the pharmacotherapy of neurological/psychiatric disorders. *The Scientific Pages of Brain Disorders*, v. 1, p. 1-3, 2017.

[273] Bergantin, LB; Caricati-Neto A. Novel challenges for the therapeutics of depression: Pharmacological modulation of interaction between

the intracellular signaling pathways mediated by Ca^{2+} and cAMP. *Journal of Addiction Therapy and Research*, v. 1, p. 1-6, 2017.

[274] Bergantin, LB; Caricati-Neto A. The 'Calcium Paradox' Due To Ca^{2+}/Camp Interaction: New Insights for the Neuroscience Field. *Journal of Neuroscience and Neurological Disorders*, v. 1, p. 12-15, 2017.

[275] Bergantin, LB; Caricati-Neto A. CCBs and neuroprotection: a genuine benefit. *Journal of pharmacology & clinical research (JPCR)*, v. 2, p. 1, 2017.

[276] Bergantin, LB; Caricati-Neto A. From a 'Eureka Insight' to Novel Concepts in Pharmaceutical Sciences: Role of $Ca^{2+/}$cAMP Intracellular Signalling Interaction. *Annals of Clinical and Laboratory Research*, v. 05, p. 1, 2017.

[277] Bergantin, LB; Caricati-Neto A. Advances for the pharmacotherapy of Parkinson's disease: Pharmacological handling of the Ca^{2+}/cAMP signaling interaction. *The Scientific Pages of Brain Disorders*, v. 1, p. 1, 2017.

[278] Bergantin, LB; Caricati-Neto A. Lessons from the Discovery of the 'Calcium Paradox' due to Ca^{2+}/cAMP Interaction. *The Scientific Pages of Neurodegenerative Disorders,* v. 1, p. 1-4, 2017.

[279] Bergantin, LB; Caricati-Neto A. A New Hope for the Therapy of Alzheimer's and Parkinson's Diseases: Pharmacological Modulation of Neural Ca^{2+}/cAMP Signaling Interaction. *Brain and Nervous System Current Research*, v. 1, p. 1, 2017.

[280] Bergantin, LB; Caricati-Neto A. New concepts for clinical pathology from Ca^{2+}/cAMP signalling interaction. *Journal of Clinical Pathology and Microbes*, v. 1, p. 1, 2017.

[281] Bergantin, LB; Caricati-Neto A. Novel concepts for neurology and medicine from the interaction between signalling pathways mediated by Ca^{2+} and cAMP:an intriguing history. *Journal of Pediatric Neurological Disorders*, v. 3, p. 1, 2017.

[282] Caricati-Neto A; Scorza FA; Scorza CA; Cysneiros RM; Rodrigues FSM; Bergantin LB. Sudden Unexpected Death in Parkinson's Disease and the Pharmacological Modulation of the Ca^{2+}/cAMP

Signaling Interaction: A Shot of Good News. *Brain Disorders & Therapy*, v. 06, p. 1, 2017.

[283] Bergantin, LB; Caricati-Neto A. Advances for the pharmacotherapy of depression - Presenting the rising star: Ca^{2+}/camp signaling interaction. *Journal of Systems and Integrative Neuroscience*, v. 3, p. 1-5, 2017.

[284] Bergantin, LB; Caricati-Neto A. From a 'eureka insight' to a novel potential therapeutic target to treat Alzheimer's disease. *Scientific Pages Alzheimer's disease*, v. 1, p. 34, 2017.

[285] Bergantin, LB; Caricati-Neto A. Emerging Concepts for Neuroscience Field from Ca^{2+}/cAMP Signalling Interaction. *Journal of Neurology and Experimental Neuroscience*, v. 03, p. 29-32, 2017.

[286] Bergantin, LB; Caricati-Neto A. Clinical Research: Good News Coming from Ca^{2+}/cAMP Signaling Interaction. *Annals of Clinical and Laboratory Research*, v. 05, p. 1, 2017.

[287] Bergantin, LB; Caricati-Neto A. Perspectives of The Pharmacological Modulation of Ca^{2+}/Camp Signaling Interaction as a New Neuroprotector Therapeutic Strategy for Amyotrophic Lateral Sclerosis (ALS). *Biomedical Journal of Scientific & Technical Research*, v. 1, p. 1, 2017.

[288] Bergantin, LB; Caricati-Neto A. Novel therapeutics from old pharmaceuticals: The Ca^{2+}/cAMP signaling interaction as a new pharmaceutical target for treatment of diseases related to aging. *Journal of Neurology and Neurodisorders*, v. 1, p. 1, 2017.

[289] Bergantin, LB; Caricati-Neto A. Pharmaceutical intervention on C^{a2+}/cAMP signaling interaction: benefits for combating neurodegeneration and diseases related to aging. *International Journal of Human Anatomy*, v. 1, p. 1, 2017.

[290] Bergantin, LB; Caricati-Neto A. A New Hope for the Therapy of the Neurodegenerative Diseases: Pharmacological Modulation of Neural Ca2+/Camp Signaling Interaction. *Journal of Pharmaceutical Research and Drug Design*, v. 1, p. e101, 2017.

[291] Dayalu, P; Albin, RL (2015) "Huntington disease: pathogenesis and treatment." *Neurologic Clinics*. 33(1): 101–14.

[292] Walker FO (2007). "Huntington's disease". *Lancet.* 369(9557): 218–28.

[293] Driver-Dunckley E, Caviness JN (2007). "Huntington's disease." In Schapira AHV. *Neurology and Clinical Neuroscience.* Mosby Elsevier. pp 879–885.

[294] Harjes P, Wanker EE (2003) "The hunt for huntingtin function: interaction partners tell many different stories." *Trends Biochem. Sci.* 28(8): 425–33.

[295] Goehler H, Lalowski M, Stelzl U, et al. (2004) "A protein interaction network links GIT1, an enhancer of Huntingtin aggregation, to Huntington's disease." *Mol. Cell.* 15(6): 853–65.

[296] Cattaneo E, Zuccato C, Tartari M (2005) "Normal huntingtin function: an alternative approach to Huntington's disease." *Nat. Rev. Neurosci.* 6(12): 919–30.

[297] Glajch, KE and Sadri-Vakili, G (2015) "Epigenetic Mechanisms Involved in Huntington's Disease Pathogenesis." *J Huntington's disease* 4(1): 1–15.

[298] Bates, Gillian P.; Dorsey, Ray; Gusella, James F.; Hayden, Michael R.; Kay, Chris; Leavitt, Blair R.; Nance, Martha; Ross, Christopher A.; Scahill, Rachael I.; Wetzel, Ronald; Wild, Edward J.; Tabrizi, Sarah J. (2015). "Huntington disease." *Nature Reviews Disease Primers:* 15005.

[299] Juntas Morales R, Pageot N, Taieb G, Camu W (2017) Adult-onset spinal muscular atrophy: An update. *Rev Neurol* (Paris). 173(5):308-319.

[300] Sommer N, Loschmann PA, Northoff GH, Weller M, Steinbrecher A, Steinbach JP et al. (1995) The antidepressant rolipram suppresses cytokine production and prevents autoimmune encephalomyelitis. *Nat Med.* 1:244–248.

[301] Xiao L, O'Callaghan JP, O'Donnell JM (2011) Effects of repeated treatment with phosphodiesterase-4 inhibitors on cAMP signaling, hippocampal cell proliferation, and behavior in the forced-swim test. *J Pharmacol Exp Ther.* 338:641–647.

[302] Hanon O, Pequignot R, Seux ML, Lenoir H et al. (2006) Relationship between antihypertensive drug therapy and cognitive function in elderly hypertensive patients with memory complaints. *J Hypertens* 24(10): 2101–2107.

[303] Onozuka H, Nakajima A, Matsuzaki K, Shin RW et al. (2008) Nobiletin, a citrus flavonoid, improves memory impairment and Abeta pathology in a transgenic mouse model of Alzheimer's disease. *J Pharmacol Exp Ther* 326(3): 739-44.

[304] De-Paula, VJ., Radanovic, M., Diniz, BS., Forlenza, OV., 2012. Alzheimer's disease. *Subcell. Biochem.* 65, 329-52.

[305] Samochocki, M., Höffle, A., Fehrenbacher, A., Jostock, R., Ludwig, J. et al. 2003. Galantamine is an allosterically potentiating ligand of neuronal nicotinic but not of muscarinic acetylcholine receptors. *J. Pharmacol. Exp. Ther.* 305, 1024-36.

[306] Li Y, Wu KJ, Yu SJ, Tamargo IA, Wang Y, Greig NH. 2016. Neurotrophic and neuroprotective effects of oxyntomodulin in neuronal cells and a rat model of stroke. *Exp Neurol.* 288: 104-113.

[307] Wild, EJ; Tabrizi, SJ. (2014) "Targets for future clinical trials in Huntington's disease: what's in the pipeline?" *Movement disorders: official journal of the Movement Disorder Society.* 29(11): 1434–45.

[308] Gines S, Seong IS, Fossale E, et al. (2003) Specific progressive cAMP reduction implicates energy deficit in presymptomatic Huntington's disease knock-in mice. *Hum Mol Genet.* 12: 497–508.

[309] Sugars KL, Brown R, Cook LJ, Swartz J, Rubinsztein DC (2004) Decreased cAMP response element-mediated transcription: an early event in exon 1 and full-length cell models of Huntington's disease that contributes to polyglutamine pathogenesis. *J Biol Chem.* 279(6): 4988-99.

[310] Mattson MP, Bezprozvanny I (2008) Neuronal Calcium Mishandling and the Pathogenesis of Alzheimer's Disease. *Trends Neurosci.* 31(9): 454-63.

[311] Guo Q (1999) Increased vulnerability of hippocampal neurons to excitotoxic necrosis in presenilin-1 mutant knock-in mice. *Nat Med.* 5:101–106.

[312] Stutzmann GE, Caccamo A, LaFerla FM, Parker I (2004) Dysregulated IP3 signaling in cortical neurons of knock-in mice expressing an Alzheimer's-linked mutation in presenilin1 results in exaggerated Ca^{2+} signals and altered membrane excitability. *J Neurosci.* 24:508–513.

[313] Mattson MP (2004) Pathways towards and away from Alzheimer's disease. *Nature.* 430:631–639.

[314] Mattson MP (1990) Antigenic changes similar to those seen in neurofibrillary tangles are elicited by glutamate and Ca^{2+} influx in cultured hippocampal neurons. *Neuron.* 4:105–117.

[315] Mattson MP, Magnus T (2006) Ageing and neuronal vulnerability. *Nat Rev Neurosci.* 7:278–294.

[316] Iadecola C, Yaffe K, Biller J, Bratzke LC, Faraci FM, Gorelick PB, et al. Impact of Hypertension on Cognitive Function. *A Scientific Statement from the American Heart Association. Hypertension* 2016;68:e67-e94.

[317] Marfany A, Sierra C, Camafort M, Doménech M, Coca A. (2018) High blood pressure, Alzheimer disease and antihypertensive treatment. *Panminerva Med* 60(1):8-16.

[318] Qiu C, Winblad B, Fratiglioni L. The age dependent relation of blood pressure to cognitive function and dementia. *Lancet Neurol* 2005;4:487-99.

[319] Kennelly S, Collins O. Walking the Cognitive "Minefield" Between High and Low Blood Pressure. *J Alzheimers Dis* 2012;32:609-21.

[320] Ashby EL, Miners JS, Kehoe PG, Love S. Effects of hypertension and anti-hypertensive treatment on amyloid-ß plaque load and Aß-synthesizing and Aß-degrading enzymes in frontal cortex. *J Alzheimers Dis* 2016;50:1191-203.

[321] Walker KA, Power MC, Gottesman RF. Defining the Relationship Between Hypertension, Cognitive Decline, and Dementia: a Review. *Curr Hypertens Rep* 2017;19:24.

[322] Langbaum JBS, Chen K, Launer LJ, Fleisher AS, Lee W, Liu X, et al. Blood pressure is associated with higher brain amyloid burden and

lower glucose metabolism in healthy late middle-age persons. *Neurobiol Aging* 2012;33:827.e11-19.

[323] Gorelick PB, Scuteri A, Black SE, Decarli C, Greenberg SM, Iadecola C, et al. Vascular contributions to cognitive impairment and dementia: a statement for healthcare professionals from the American Heart Association/American Stroke Association. *Stroke* 2011;42:2672-713.

[324] Rouch L, Cestac P, Hanon O, Cool C, Helmer C, Bouhanick B, et al. Antihypertensive Drugs, Prevention of Cognitive Decline and Dementia: A Systematic Review of Observational Studies, Randomized Controlled Trials and Meta-Analyses, with Discussion of Potential Mechanisms. *CNS Drugs* 2015;29:113-30.

[325] Forette F, Seux ML, Staessen JA, Thijs L, Birkenhäger WH, Babarskiene MR, et al. Prevention of dementia in randomised double-blind placebo-controlled Systolic Hypertension in Europe (Syst-Eur) trial. *Lancet* 1998;352:1347-51.

[326] Bari M Di, Pahor M, Franse LV, Shorr RI, Wan JY, Ferrucci L, et al. Dementia and Disability Outcomes in Large Hypertension Trials: Lessons Learned from the Systolic Hypertension in the Elderly Program (SHEP) Trial. *Am J Epidemiol* 2001;153:72-8.

[327] Weycker D, Nichols GA, O'Keeffe-Rosetti M, Edelsberg J, Vincze G, Khan ZM, Oster G. (2009) Excess risk of diabetes in persons with hypertension. *Diabetes Complications.* 23(5):330-6.

[328] Bernard MYC, Chao L (2012) Diabetes and Hypertension: Is There a Common Metabolic Pathway? *Curr Atheroscler Rep* 14(2): 160–166.

[329] Cheung BM. The hypertension-diabetes continuum. *J Cardiovasc Pharmacol.* 2010; 55: 333–9.

[330] Landsberg L, Molitch M. Diabetes and hypertension: pathogenesis, prevention and treatment. *Clin Exp Hypertens.* 2004;26:621–628. doi: 10.1081/CEH-200031945.

[331] Gress TW, Nieto FJ, Shahar E, et al. Hypertension and antihypertensive therapy as risk factors for type 2 diabetes mellitus. Atherosclerosis Risk in Communities Study. *N Engl J Med.* 2000;342:905–912. doi: 10.1056/NEJM200003303421301.

[332] Cheung BM, Wat NM, Tso AW, et al. Association between raised blood pressure and dysglycemia in Hong Kong Chinese. *Diabetes Care.* 2008;31:1889–1891. doi: 10.2337/dc08-0405.

[333] Yulia K, Anath S, Stuart JF, April PC, Monika MS (2016) Calcium channel blocker use is associated with lower fasting serum glucose among adults with diabetes from the REGARDS study. *Diabetes Res Clin Pract.* 115: 115–121.

[334] Xu G, Chen J, Jing G, Shalev A. Preventing beta-cell loss and diabetes with calcium channel blockers. *Diabetes.* 2012;61(4):848–56.

[335] Mccrimmon RJ, Ryan CM, Frier BM. Diabetes and cognitive dysfunction. *Lancet.* 2012;379(9833):2291–2299.

[336] Munshi M, Grande L, Hayes M, et al. Cognitive dysfunction is associated with poor diabetes control in older adults. *Diabetes Care.* 2006;29(8):1794–1799.

[337] Sinclair AJ, Girling AJ, Bayer AJ. Cognitive dysfunction in older subjects with diabetes mellitus: impact on diabetes self-management and use of care services. All Wales Research into Elderly (AWARE) Study. *Diabetes Res Clin Pract.* 2000;50(3):203–212.

[338] Alencar RC, Cobas RA, Gomes MB. Assessment of cognitive status in patients with type 2 diabetes through the mini-mental status examination: a cross-sectional study. *Diabetol Metab Syndr.* 2010;2(1):10.

[339] Wessels AM, Lane KA, Gao S, Hall KS, Unverzagt FW, Hendrie HC. Diabetes and cognitive decline in elderly African Americans: a 15-year follow-up study. *Alzheimers Demen.* 2011;7(4):418–424.

[340] Feinkohl I, Keller M, Robertson CM, et al. Clinical and subclinical macrovascular disease as predictors of cognitive decline in older patients with type 2 diabetes: the Edinburgh type 2 diabetes study. *Diabetes Care.* 2013;36(9):2779–2786.

[341] Zhao Q, Roberts RO, Ding D, et al. Diabetes is associated with worse executive function in both Eastern and Western populations: Shanghai aging study and mayo clinic study of aging. *J Alzheimers Dis.* 2015;47(1):167–176.

[342] Qiu C, Sigurdsson S, Zhang Q, et al. Diabetes, markers of brain pathology and cognitive function. *Ann Neurol.* 2014;75(1):138–146.

[343] Moran C, Phan TG, Chen J, et al. Brain atrophy in type 2 diabetes: regional distribution and influence on cognition. *Diabetes Care.* 2013;36(12):4036–4042.

[344] Kooistra M, Geerlings MI, van der Graaf Y, et al. Vascular brain lesions, brain atrophy, and cognitive decline. The Second Manifestations of ARTerial disease–magnetic resonance (SMART-MR) study. *Neurobiol Aging.* 2014;35(1):35–41.

[345] van Elderen SG, de Roos A, de Craen AJ, et al. Progression of brain atrophy and cognitive decline in diabetes mellitus: a 3-year follow-up. *Neurology.* 2010;75(11):997–1002.

[346] Bruce DG, Casey GP, Grange V, et al. Cognitive impairment, physical disability and depressive symptoms in older diabetic patients: the Fre-mantle Cognition in Diabetes Study. *Diabetes Res Clin Pract.* 2003;61(1):59–67.

[347] Watson GS, Craft S. The role of insulin resistance in the pathogenesis of Alzheimer's disease: implications for treatment. *CNS Drugs.* 2003;17(1):27–45.

[348] Kodl CT, Seaquist ER. Cognitive dysfunction and diabetes mellitus. *Endocr Rev.* 2008;29(4):494–511.

[349] Cunnane S, Nugent S, Roy M, et al. Brain fuel metabolism, aging, and Alzheimer's disease. *Nutrition.* 2011;27(1):3–20. doi:10.1016/j.nut.2010.07.021.

[350] Cunnane SC, Plourde M, Pifferi F, Bégin M, Féart C, Barberger-Gateau P. Fish, docosahexaenoic acid and Alzheime's disease. *Prog Lipid Res.* 2009;48(5):239–256. doi:10.1016/j.plipres.2009.04.001.

[351] Aliev G, Shahida K, Gan SH, et al. Alzheimer disease and type 2 diabetes mellitus: the link to tyrosine hydroxylase and probable nutritional strategies. *CNS Neurol Disord Drug Targets.* 2014;13(3):467–477. doi:10.2174/18715273113126660153.

[352] Siew Hua G, Kamal MA, Lima MM, Khalil MI, Pasupuleti VR, Aliev G. Medicinal plants in management of type 2 diabetes and

neurodegenerative disorders. *Evid Based Complement Alternat Med.* 2015;2015:686872. doi:10.1155/2015/686872.

[353] Errante PR, Caricati-Neto A, Bergantin LB (2017) Insights for the inhibition of cancer progression: Revisiting Ca^{2+} and cAMP signalling pathways. *Adv Cancer Prevention* 2: e103.

[354] PR Errante, S Francisco, A Caricati-Neto, Bergantin LB (2017) The Pharmacological Modulation of Ca^{2+}/Camp Intracellular Signaling Pathways and Traditional Antitumoral Pharmaceuticals. *Journal of Clinical & Experimental Oncology* 6:4.

[355] PR Errante, AA Leite, FS Menezes-Rodrigues, A Caricati-Neto, Bergantin LB (2017) A novel potential therapeutic target as adjuvant treatment for cancer: the pharmacological interference on the Ca2+/cAMP cellular signaling pathways. *Enliven: Chall Cancer Detec Ther* 1, 1-2.

[356] PR Errante, FS Menezes-Rodrigues, AA Leite, A Caricati-Neto, Bergantin LB (2017) The second messengers Ca^{2+} and cAMP as potential therapeutic targets for the control of cancer progression. *Adv Cancer Prev* 2, 1-2.

[357] Caricati-Neto A, Bergantin LB (2017) Pharmacological modulation of neural Ca^{2+}/camp signaling interaction as therapeutic goal for treatment of Alzheimer's disease. *J Syst Integr Neurosci* 3: doi:10.15761/JSIN.1000185.

[358] Caricati-Neto A, Bergantin LB (2017) The passion of a scientific discovery: the "calcium paradox" due to Ca2+/camp interaction. *J Syst Integr Neurosci* 3: doi:10.15761/JSIN.1000186.

[359] Caricati-Neto A, Bergantin LB (2017) From a "eureka insight" to a novel potential therapeutic target to treat Parkinson's disease: The Ca^{2+}/camp signalling interaction. *J Syst Integr Neurosci* 4: doi:10.15761/JSIN.1000187.

ABOUT THE AUTHOR

Dr. Leandro Bueno Bergantin, PhD, received his academic education at EPM-UNIFESP (Brazil): biomedicine (2008), MSc (2010) and PhD (2014); with a research visiting period in UAM (Spain). His research involves cell signalling mediated by Ca^{2+} and cAMP, including its role in neuropsychopharmacology, autonomic and cardiovascular pharmacology, and cancer. Dr. Bergantin's research work solved the enigma of the paradoxical effects produced by L-type Ca^{2+} channel blockers (CCB), which was published in *Cell Calcium* (JCR: 4.87) and achieved the position 'ScienceDirect TOP 25 Hottest Articles' (ranked #1 on the TOP 25 for *Cell Calcium*, 2013). This discovery generated 17 articles published in international journals indexed in PubMed, in which 14 of them Dr. Bergantin is the sole author, e.g., *Cancer Letters* (JCR: 7.36), *Pharmacological Research* (JCR: 5.89), *Current Protein & Peptide Science* (JCR: 2.52), *Current Pharmaceutical Design* (JCR: 2.20), *Psychiatry Research* (JCR: 2.11), *Anti-Cancer Agents in Medicinal Chemistry* (JCR: 2.04). Briefly, since 1975 several clinical and experimental studies have reported that acute and chronic administration of L-type CCB, such as nifedipine, produces reduction in arterial pressure associated with a paradoxical increase of sympathetic activity. In 2013, Dr. Bergantin discovered that this paradoxical increase in sympathetic activity produced by L-type CCB is due to the interaction of Ca^{2+}/cAMP signalling, then opening new avenues for biomedical research, e.g., neurological and psychiatry diseases, cancer, diabetes, and asthma. Dr. Bergantin is member of several editorial boards of international journals, and has been frequently invited to be honorable guest in international conferences as well as to participating in media interviews.

INDEX

A

aging, 41, 56, 60, 61, 77, 78, 82, 84, 88, 89, 90, 93, 102, 106, 143, 147, 148, 149
amyloid cascade, 84, 139
amyloid plaques, 79, 93, 94
amyloidogenesis, 84, 85
amyotrophic lateral sclerosis, xv, 40, 46, 60, 105, 139, 140, 143
antihypertensive therapy, 1, 54, 55, 57, 58, 61, 62, 66, 67, 73, 94, 114, 116, 147
arterial pressure, 1, 54, 57, 66, 73, 107, 113, 151
ATP and noradrenaline, 11

B

Bergantin, iii, 3, 4, 8, 13, 32, 34, 56, 65, 116, 132, 135, 140, 141, 142, 143, 150, 151

C

Ca2+ and cAMP, 7, 9, 13, 33, 47, 53, 57, 66, 71, 107, 108, 112, 113, 114, 142, 150, 151
Ca2+ entry and cAMP, 5
Ca2+ signalling, vii, 7, 13, 18, 19, 24, 30, 77, 81, 82, 87, 91, 109
Ca2+/cAMP interaction, 4, 6, 7, 9, 10, 34, 40, 73, 74, 75, 105, 141, 142, 150
Ca2+/cAMP signalling interaction, 47, 53, 54, 56, 57, 58, 59, 62, 65, 66, 67, 68, 70, 72, 75, 95, 99, 107, 108, 112, 113, 114, 142, 150
calcium paradox, 5, 6, 7, 9, 11, 13, 33, 40, 54, 57, 66, 105, 107, 112, 113, 116, 141, 142, 150
cAMP levels, 5, 7, 33, 52, 109
catecholamine release, 8, 9, 10, 11, 21, 29, 118, 120, 123, 137
cellular communication, 15
chromaffin cells, 6, 8, 9, 10, 11, 12, 13, 14, 16, 17, 18, 19, 20, 21, 22, 23, 24, 25, 26, 27, 28, 29, 31, 32, 33, 35, 36, 58, 67, 117, 118, 119, 120, 121, 122, 123, 124,

125, 126, 127, 128, 129, 130, 131, 137, 138, 139

D

depression, 9, 32, 40, 43, 44, 45, 46, 50, 52, 71, 86, 102, 105, 106, 141, 143
diabetes, i, iii, viii, xi, xvi, 59, 74, 91, 97, 98, 99, 101, 102, 104, 125, 133, 134, 147, 148, 149, 152
diltiazem, 1, 2, 72, 112
dopamine loss, 42

E

exocytosis, vii, 9, 10, 12, 13, 15, 16, 17, 18, 19, 20, 21, 22, 24, 27, 28, 29, 31, 32, 34, 35, 36, 52, 53, 57, 66, 75, 105, 117, 118, 119, 121, 123, 124, 125, 126, 128, 129, 130, 131, 132, 135, 137, 138, 139

F

forskolin, 3, 4, 5, 9, 10, 36, 72, 118, 119, 123

H

healthy brain aging, 90
hypertension, i, iii, viii, xi, 11, 54, 57, 59, 66, 74, 93, 94, 95, 97, 98, 99, 120, 146, 147

I

IBMX, xv, 3, 4, 5, 10, 36, 72
insulin levels, 99
intracellular messengers, 13, 18, 30, 32, 51

M

memory dysfunctions, 101
mitochondria, xv, 20, 21, 78, 120, 122, 126, 127, 129, 130

N

neurodegeneration, 39, 50, 102, 143
neurofibrillary tangles, 83, 93, 146
neurological and psychiatric disorders, 37, 39, 40, 55, 56, 71, 75, 105, 108, 114, 116, 140, 141
neuroprotection, 52, 62, 74, 105, 108, 113, 141, 142
nifedipine, 1, 5, 6, 9, 11, 57, 58, 66, 67, 72, 73, 74, 116, 151
nifedipine paradoxical effect, 9
Nobel Prize in Physiology or Medicine, 20
nutraceuticals, 104

P

PDE inhibitors, 10, 69, 75, 105
pharmacological manipulation, xii, 14, 73, 74

R

rolipram, ix, 3, 4, 5, 7, 8, 9, 10, 36, 55, 58, 62, 67, 70, 72, 73, 74, 106, 114, 144

S

secretory machine, 16, 132
smooth muscles, 2, 4, 5, 112, 116
spinal muscular atrophy, xvi, 40, 53, 56, 57, 144
stimulus-secretion coupling, 19, 121, 126, 134

sympathetic hyperactivity, 1, 11, 54, 57, 58, 66, 67, 73, 107, 113

sympathetic neurons, 1, 11, 12, 13, 16, 17, 18, 20, 23, 30, 33, 54, 58, 67, 107, 113

synaptic vesicles, xvi, 16, 132

verapamil, ix, 1, 2, 3, 4, 5, 6, 7, 8, 9, 57, 66, 72, 73, 106, 111, 112, 116, 117

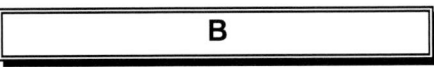

β-amyloid peptide, 40, 61

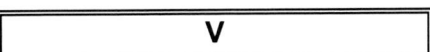

vascular dementia, xvi, 40, 59, 102